Supporting Parents and Families with Perinatal Mental Health and Wellbeing

of related interest

Postnatal PTSD
A Guide for Health Professionals
Kim Thomas with Shona McCann
ISBN 978 1 78775 620 5
eISBN 978 1 78775 621 2

Supporting Fat Birth
A Book for Birth Professionals and Parents
AJ Silver
ISBN 978 1 83997 633 9
eISBN 978 1 83997 634 6

Supporting Queer Birth
A Book for Birth Professionals and Parents
AJ Silver
ISBN 978 1 83997 045 0
eISBN 978 1 83997 046 7

Supporting Autistic People Through Pregnancy and Childbirth
Hayley Morgan, Emma Durman and Karen Henry
Forewords by Carly Jones, Wenn B. Lawson and Sheena Byrom
ISBN 978 1 83997 105 1
eISBN 978 1 83997 106 8

SUPPORTING PARENTS and FAMILIES with PERINATAL MENTAL HEALTH and WELLBEING

An Introduction for Professionals

Dr Jane Hanley
and **Mark Williams**

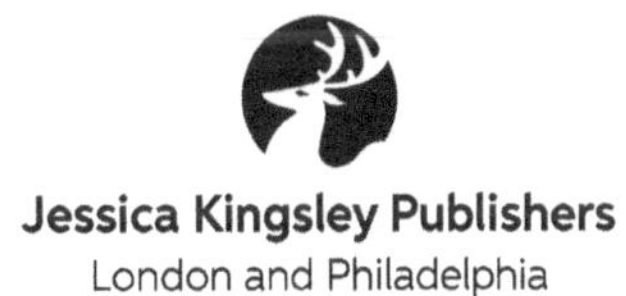

Jessica Kingsley Publishers
London and Philadelphia

First published in Great Britain in 2026 by Jessica Kingsley Publishers
An imprint of John Murray Press

2

A CIP catalogue record for this title is available from the British Library and the Library of Congress.

ISBN 978 1 83997 037 5
eISBN 978 1 83997 038 2

Printed and bound in the United States by Integrated Books International

Jessica Kingsley Publishers' policy is to use papers that are natural, renewable and recyclable products and made from wood grown in sustainable forests. The logging and manufacturing processes are expected to conform to the environmental regulations of the country of origin.

Jessica Kingsley Publishers
Carmelite House
50 Victoria Embankment
London EC4Y 0DZ

www.jkp.com

John Murray Press
Part of Hodder & Stoughton Limited
An Hachette UK Company

The authorized representative in the EEA is Hachette Ireland, 8 Castlecourt Centre, Dublin 15, D15 XTP3, Ireland (email: info@hbgi.ie)

Contents

CHAPTER 1

Introduction

WHAT IS PERINATAL MENTAL HEALTH?

The term 'perinatal' refers to the period of time around childbirth. Interpretations of the timeframe of this period vary; in some cases, it includes the time before conception until two years after an infant has been born. In the UK, the First 1001 Days Movement raises awareness of the developmental significance of the first two and a half years of a child's life.[1]

Research indicates that becoming a parent can be a transformative experience; a study by Babetin (2020) suggests that the transition to motherhood is a psychologically profound experience that both overlaps with and is distinct from the physical experience of becoming a mother. Parenthood can be life-changing. It is exhausting, stressful and demanding, but also joyful, illuminating and heart-warming. It can have a dramatic impact on relationships, work–life balance and emotional wellbeing. Relationships may undergo challenging adjustments to enable parents to accept a new infant into the family. Work arrangements may have to be restructured to accommodate the infant's needs, whilst the emotional journey for both parents can be educational and enlightening.

As the 'perinatal period' has only in recent years been widely used as a clinical term, some parents are unsure exactly what it

1 https://parentinfantfoundation.org.uk/1001-days

means. In this guide, we consider the period to start at conception and end two years following the birth of the infant. This guide focuses on mental health during the entire perinatal period. It addresses the importance of supporting the mental and emotional wellbeing of families at this important time, and it provides valuable information about the many mental health conditions that may affect parents before and after the birth of their child(ren). Our emphasis is on promoting the wellbeing of the whole family – mothers, fathers and children – and enabling parents to better understand and manage their mental health.

Pregnancy and childbirth can be a time of joy for parents and the wider family and community: a period when a new baby is eagerly anticipated and welcomed. Professionals encourage parents to take care of themselves and their developing foetus. Mothers are advised to follow a nutritious diet and avoid alcohol or other potentially harmful substances, while the value of a low-stress lifestyle and robust social and economic support are emphasised. However, ideal pregnancy and childbirth scenarios are often not the reality. It is not always easy for parents to comply with all the recommendations practitioners provide in the perinatal period, particularly when they are experiencing adverse conditions.

Many mental health conditions can affect parents during the perinatal period, and these conditions can arise at any time during pregnancy and after childbirth.

This chapter provides a brief introduction to some of the most common mental health conditions and provides information on what parents may experience at this time. Parental mental health problems often occur alongside stressful life experiences, such as pregnancy and birth. More detailed information about these conditions can be found in subsequent chapters.

COMMON CONDITIONS IN THE PERINATAL PERIOD

Anxiety can manifest in several different forms, and symptoms sometimes overlap across conditions. Some of the major anxiety-related conditions, or conditions where anxiety is a symptom, are:

- generalised anxiety
- social anxiety disorder
- obsessive compulsive disorder
- post-traumatic stress disorder.

We will also discuss eating disorders in this section.

Generalised anxiety

Generalised anxiety is common: various studies suggest that anxiety occurs in one in four parents, but this data only reflects self-reported or clinically diagnosed cases (Mental Health Foundation, 2020; National Institute of Mental Health, 2024; WHO 2001). In the perinatal period, anxiety can present in many guises: a parent may be anxious about the development of their unborn infant or feel uncomfortable going out in public; it may manifest as a phobia, an obsession, an eating disorder, or through addiction or self-harm. Symptoms are physical, emotional and behavioural, ranging from a parent suffering palpitations and irritability to experiencing digestion problems, difficulties concentrating or feelings of anger.

Social anxiety disorder

According to a 2017 US study, social anxiety disorder affects an estimated 8% of women and 6% of men (National Comorbidity Survey, 2017). This condition may affect parents, particularly if they have a history of anxiety or of feeling uncomfortable in social situations. Some people living with this condition can experience excessive worry and guilt in social contexts. Social anxiety can exacerbate feelings of low self-esteem; people with social anxiety often fear being humiliated due to being perceived as socially inadequate, boring or of little interest to others. These overpowering doubts can produce all the symptoms of anxiety, and for some people these feelings become so uncomfortable that they completely avoid any social situations (Deklava *et al.*, 2015). If social anxiety disorder is not recognised and treated, there is a risk that it may lead to depression.

Obsessive compulsive disorder (OCD)

OCD is characterised by three main parts:

- 'Obsessions – frequent unpleasant thoughts, images, urges or doubts
- Anxiety – distress caused by these unpleasant thoughts
- Compulsions – behaviours like washing hands or mental acts such as counting, that the person keeps repeating, to try to reduce their anxiety or to prevent bad things from happening.' (Wales Mental Health Network, 2023)

Some research indicates that 8% of mothers experience OCD during pregnancy and 17% experience it postnatally in the first ten months following childbirth (Fairbrother *et al.*, 2021). There are some studies showing OCD affecting fathers in the perinatal period (Chen, Schultz & Hughes, 2024). Some behaviours indicating that a parent is suffering from OCD might not be visible to professionals, making the condition challenging to recognise.

Providing professional support can help the parent. OCD is treatable. Usually, it is treated with CBT and sometimes additionally or solely with medication. Cognitive behavioural therapy (CBT) with exposure and response prevention is cited by Mind as the recommended treatment.

Post-traumatic stress disorder (PTSD)

The symptoms of PTSD, caused by witnessing or experiencing a traumatic event, include intrusive memories, emotional numbing and hypervigilance. Parents with PTSD may experience nightmares, mood swings that are more frequently negative than positive and panic attacks (Stuijfzand, Garthus-Niegel & Horsch, 2020). Disturbed sleep from frequent nightmares and intense dreams is common in PTSD as the brain struggles to assimilate and process traumatic experiences. This can reduce parents' ability to rest and elevate their anxiety levels (Lancel *et al.*, 2021). Traumatic births can profoundly affect the mental health of mothers (Beck. Watson & Gable, 2018). Maternity staff should ensure that mothers are thoroughly debriefed and made aware of the rationale for procedures during childbirth as well as details of the outcomes. For fathers, cases of birth-related PTSD have been largely under-reported, and evidence that fathers also experience anxiety, PTSD and depression during the perinatal period has emerged only relatively recently (Daniels, Arden-Close & Mayers, 2020; Vischer *et al.*, 2020).

Debriefing for a traumatic birth

Following a traumatic birth, it is difficult to know when it is the right time to debrief or to ask the parents how they are feeling and whether they are okay.

For some parents, a debrief is welcome; for others, it might be too soon to think too deeply about their experience. A debrief is usually a structured conversation by a health practitioner, which allows the mother who has experienced a traumatic birth to discuss her thoughts and feelings about the birth, to understand what decisions were made, and why, and more importantly to have the opportunity to ask questions. The parent may need to validate their experience and to resolve any feeling they may have of self-blame or guilt.

If appropriate, the health practitioner can offer practical support or refer the mother or parent to a more specialised service. Whether a full psychological debriefing is useful, is open to debate, as there seems to be a lack of evidence about whether this is effective. It tends not to prevent a further occurrence of PTSD or reduce any psychological stress, and some studies have suggested that psychological debriefing may have the potential to cause further harm (Bastos *et al.*, 2015). Less-structured midwife-led debriefing is highly variable, so it is difficult to say whether the evidence on psychological debriefing might apply there too (McKenzie-McHarg *et al.*, 2015).

However, despite the lack of evidence, many parents have reported that they would like to discuss their experience of the birth and find comfort and value in having their questions about the decisions made answered. Demonstrating care and compassion after a traumatic event is sometimes all that parents need, and if the health practitioner feels that the needs are not met, then collaborating with other services is often helpful (Collins, 2006).

Eating disorders

Eating disorders include bulimia, which involves eating excessive amounts of food to the point of experiencing considerable discomfort or pain, and anorexia, a condition associated with extreme dieting and sometimes induced starvation to attain or maintain a perceived ideal body weight. Some parents may have a history of an eating disorder but have managed to control it prior to the pregnancy. Weight gain during this period can sometimes cause a mother significant distress as she may feel she is gaining too much weight, but she also understands that altering her diet can have consequences for her unborn child. Sometimes, parents may change their eating habits in an attempt to make themselves feel better, more relaxed and able to cope, but making such adjustments can have damaging consequences for not only their mental and physical health, but that of their unborn child (Abraham, 2016).

Bigorexia nervosa

We are becoming more aware of lesser-known (and not always clinically recognised) conditions that are associated with the perinatal period. One example of a condition about which we have increased awareness is often termed 'bigorexia'.

Bigorexia nervosa, a body dysmorphic disorder (or sometimes

considered an eating disorder), is now a commonly used term to describe the image some people may have of their body shape, particularly if they are used to regularly going to the gym to get fit and to develop a muscular physique. Bigorexia nervosa was initially reported in male bodybuilders, who continually ruminated about their body mass and being larger or more muscular (Mosley, 2009). However, researchers found that this behaviour was not just confined to bodybuilders, but also to the general population. It was found that those who had bigorexia nervosa shared the same symptoms as those who were diagnosed with anorexia nervosa, as they were concerned with their body weight and shape (Murray *et al.*, 2012).

It is important to understand that what some may feel is a mild anxiety can sometimes develop into a mental health disorder.

Symptoms of bigorexia may include excessively concentrating on lifting heavier weights and using anabolic steroids or other performance-enhancing drugs. Someone experiencing bigorexia might assess their physique in mirrors, feeling dissatisfied unless they meet rigorous goals.

For many parents, caring for an infant prevents them from regularly attending the gym. This can lead to a decline in physical and mental fitness and, significantly, in their satisfaction with their body. The parent may resent not being able to train as they used to and become increasingly aware of and upset by what they perceive to be their deteriorating physique. As a result of this increased anxiety state, they may start to avoid social situations where their body will be exposed, such as a swimming pool or the beach. It may also mean they will wear clothing that will not emphasise their shape (Vasiliu, 2023).

As there is a growing interest in staying fit and muscular, there is the possibility of an increase in the prevalence of body dysmorphia. Women who feel that they have to regain their pre-pregnancy body shape might not fully succeed, and their perceived feelings of failure may add to their level of anxiety.

Another condition relating to body image is orthorexia, 'an unhealthy obsession with eating "pure" food' (BEAT Eating Disorders, n.d.). It is not currently recognised clinically as an eating disorder.

DEPRESSION DURING THE PERINATAL PERIOD

Like anxiety, depression can present differently from person to person, and some signs and symptoms are more severe than others. Common types of depressive emotions or depression during the perinatal period are:

- the 'baby blues'
- antenatal depression
- postnatal depression.

The 'baby blues'

In the past, the 'baby blues' were often considered to be a typical stage a few days after childbirth when many mothers felt emotionally overwhelmed and tearful. It was generally assumed that these intense feelings would pass, but there is now greater awareness that, for some women, the baby blues may represent a continuation of their pre-existing symptoms of anxiety and depression (Henshaw, 2000; Moyo & Djoda, 2020) It is important for practitioners to be vigilant and observe the length and severity of the condition.

Antenatal depression

Studies have shown that two thirds of mothers who are depressed in the postnatal period had signs of depression during their pregnancy (Heron *et al.*, 2004). However, this data does not demonstrate the extent to which depression is recognised, managed or treated throughout the perinatal period.

Risk factors for antenatal depression include experiencing trauma, which may be environmental or social, financial difficulties, domestic abuse or any factors that may cause significant stress over a long period. There is overwhelming evidence suggesting that antenatally an unplanned pregnancy is a major risk factor for suicide (Legazpi *et al.*, 2022), particularly for adolescents: the risk for adolescents is over five times greater than the overall rate for women who die by suicide during pregnancy (Lindahl, Pearson & Colpe, 2005).

Symptoms range from mild, when a parent may feel sad and lonely, to severe, when a parent's mood is so low that they experience a loss of feelings and suicidal ideation.

Postnatal depression

Studies have found that one in seven mothers and one in ten fathers suffer from postnatal depression (Bergstrom, 2013; Carlberg, Edhborg & Lindberg, 2018; Carlson *et al.*, 2022). Risk factors are similar to those found in the antenatal period and might include a previous history of depression or anxiety, social isolation, domestic abuse, relationship difficulties, financial worries, the death or loss of a supportive figure, environmental disasters, or war trauma. Concern over the health of the new infant can also be a contributing factor. A family history of suicide is an indicator for postnatal depression, and there is an increased risk of suicide in mothers whose own mothers were suicidal.

As common postnatal depression symptoms include low levels of interest and joy, it can be challenging for parents experiencing postnatal depression to find sufficient energy and enthusiasm to enable them to care for their child. Postnatal depression interferes with behavioural and emotional exchanges between the parent and the infant: a mother may find it difficult to engage with her infant and to express warmth and pleasure, which is reflected in the tone of her voice or the way she holds the infant (Milgrom & Holt, 2014).

SEVERE PERINATAL MENTAL HEALTH CONDITIONS

While any condition may become severe, there are forms of mental illness that can occur in the perinatal period that often require specialist support from perinatal mental health services due to severe symptoms. In these cases, the behaviour of the parent may be a cause for concern as they may be a danger to themselves and their infant. It is important that these conditions are recognised early and that the parent, particularly the mother, has rapid access to clinical treatments. These conditions include:

- bipolar disorder
- puerperal or postpartum psychosis.

Bipolar disorder

The key features of bipolar disorder are the ways in which the moods present. Those with the disorder can have alternating episodes of:

- depression – feeling very low and lethargic
- mania – feeling very high and overactive.

Some mothers may not have previously experienced any symptoms of bipolar disorder until they became pregnant. Until recently, little was known about this condition, which primarily affects the brain and causes severe shifts in mood function. When it is at its most severe, bipolar disorder can cause episodes of extreme mania, during which a parent may have extremely high energy levels. Parents experiencing a manic period of bipolar disorder may be garrulous, speaking quickly and forming random, unconnected sentences that may signal disorganised thought processes. The content of their speech may be superficial and disjointed, and they may be easily distracted and unable to concentrate for long periods. Someone experiencing a manic episode can become irritable or aggressive if people struggle to understand them when they are unable to communicate clearly.

Puerperal psychosis

Puerperal psychosis is at the severe end of the spectrum of mental illnesses. The condition is rare and is serious and frightening for both the mother and her family (Raza & Raza, 2022). It affects one to two in 1000 mothers (Perry *et al.*, 2021). In some cases, the severity of the onset of the illness means that the mother needs immediate hospitalisation in either a psychiatric ward or, ideally, in a mother and baby unit. The mother may present a danger to herself and to her infant. Puerperal psychosis usually develops a few days following the birth, but cases do occur up to three months postnatally.

The illness can present with a distortion of the five senses, which may include visual and or auditory hallucinations, tasting, feeling or smelling things that are not actually present. Sometimes, delusions may be present, which can result in bizarre and unreal beliefs, such as the infant is not hers, or someone is trying to abduct the infant. These symptoms can be frightening and cause confusion and fear, which may result in noticeable changes in behaviours, which can cause concerns for both the mother and the partner.

HOW DO PERINATAL MENTAL HEALTH CONDITIONS AFFECT INFANTS AND CHILDREN?

As the NSPCC (2024) states: 'Many parents with mental health problems are able to give their children safe and loving care, without their children being negatively affected in any way'. However, if not well managed, the perinatal mental health conditions outlined in this chapter can profoundly affect infants and children, underlining the importance of early intervention and effective support.

There can be significant emotional and behavioural difficulties for the child of a depressed mother if the mother's depression is not adequately managed. Therefore, practitioners must recognise the condition with concern, prioritising treatment and management to ensure that families have better outcomes. Depression in fathers can also have significant impacts. Some studies have found that postnatal depression in fathers is linked to behavioural and emotional problems in their children at three-and-a-half and seven years old (Letourneau *et al.*, 2019; Nath *et al.*, 2016). One study found that fathers' depression affected their teenage daughters; some daughters of fathers with depression presented with emotional problems, particularly at around 18 years old (Gutierrez-Galve *et al.*, 2019).

Social anxiety in parents can lead to loneliness as they isolate themselves from family and other parents. This can have damaging effects on the parent's relationships with others but may also have a detrimental influence on the wellbeing of the infant, because they are denied the opportunity to socialise with others.

The distorted perception of body image associated with the eating disorders anorexia and bulimia can lead parents to believe they need to lose further weight despite being pregnant or, post-delivery, breastfeeding. It is likely that these disorders will have consequences for both the mother's and the infant's physical and mental health, as it is possible the parent will also present with anxiety or depressive symptoms, or both.

Bipolar disorder can particularly impact a mother's interaction with her infant during the first year of life, potentially leading to developmental risks (Boekhorst *et al.*, 2021). Some mothers may, initially, find it difficult to bond with their infant because of their increased fears of failure, as well as their feelings of insecurity. Some of the characteristics of the mother's mood disorder, her facial expressions and tone of voice, can make it difficult for the infant to understand her cues. Breastfeeding rates are significantly lower for bipolar mothers, and this lack of contact also has implications for bonding. Some studies have found that the children of bipolar mothers are more likely to have ADHD, anxiety and depressive symptoms (Alptekin *et al.*, 2022; Bastos *et al.*, 2022; Chang *et al.*, 2003).

It is important to recognise if someone has bipolar disorder, as if left undiagnosed, it may have long-term consequences for the infant and family. Therefore, it is essential that help and support are established as early as possible. There may be concerns from the family about the mother's mental health, particularly when she has an episode where she is unusually overactive or excited. The GP can help to support the mother and the family and may refer the mother to a specialist perinatal mental health service. There are positive measures designed to help the family, including medications aimed at treating the mother's symptoms and early interventions designed to address the needs of the mother to help her bond with her infant.

Following the culmination of the exhausting signs that a mother experiencing puerperal psychosis may express, the beliefs she communicates may be acted upon. These beliefs are sometimes about her infant; she may be convinced that the infant is not her own and that she was given the wrong baby at the hospital or, in more extreme cases, that the baby is the devil and needs to be destroyed (NHS Wales, 2022). These delusions and sometimes (though not often) actions can have serious consequences for the safeguarding of the infant.

PRACTICAL GUIDANCE FOR SUPPORTING WELLBEING IN FAMILIES BEFORE AND DURING PREGNANCY

Lifestyle behaviours and stressors have a significant influence on perinatal wellbeing; where possible, practitioners should discuss these with parents-to-be prior to conception. It is often the mother from whom the health and social care services will take a history, both ante- and postnatally, of their lifestyle and welfare.

Planning pregnancy

In some cases, where the parents already have one child, the parents' thoughts on the suitability of the timing of becoming pregnant again can be discussed. Those wishing to conceive should be encouraged to maintain or attain a healthy weight by exploring healthy lifestyle choices, such as eating regular nutritious meals and avoiding the use of alcohol and illicit drugs.

During pregnancy

Discussing and sharing resources about suitable food should be encouraged, as well as examining eating habits at various times of the week and reflecting on which moods prompt the type of food consumed. Where required, parents' alcohol intake should also be closely monitored, particularly if in the past the parent has resorted to using alcohol as a coping mechanism. Illicit substances should be avoided too; it is helpful to speak to parents about any previous drug use, as it may provide practitioners with insights into parents' coping strategies.

Exercise, sleep hygiene and stress

The importance of maintaining physical exercise should be emphasised to parents. It can be tempting to physically relax once pregnancy is established, but continuing to keep fit can help to ensure a safer delivery and promote a healthy mindset. The amount of quality sleep a parent can achieve is also significant as it can affect mood, stress levels and cognitive function.

Talking with parents about the harm that stress that can cause to the mother and the unborn child can be a constructive way to highlight any current risk factors that may exacerbate stress or even induce a stressful situation. It may help parents to open up about stress they are experiencing. If the mother experiences very stressful situations, these can activate the HPA axis (hypothalamic–pituitary–adrenal axis), which in turn triggers the release of stress hormones. Ordinarily, these are necessary to help the body cope with any impending challenges; however, too much of the stress hormone released by the mother can cross over the placenta and affect the developing foetus (Glover *et al.*, 2018). It is not always easy to prevent the pressures of daily living, but assessing the rapidity of how situations could change or why may be the first steps to alleviating some of the difficulties which may later arise.

Inclusive care during the perinatal period

In the past, it may have been assumed that the carers or parents of the infant are a mother (female) and a father (male), but families are more complex than this, and it is important to be sensitive to the different families you support. Families may include same-sex partners, paternal or maternal parents or grandparents, a partner who is not the biological parent of the infant or adoptive parents. The family may be a single parent and child. Although adoptive parents do not have the same physical experiences as birth mothers, they can feel similar emotional and mental stresses when caring for their new infant. Same-sex partners feel excluded from some services and classes, as many antenatal classes centre on heterosexual couples' experiences. A woman whose female partner is pregnant may feel excluded from the biological experience of becoming a mother, where classes such as pregnancy yoga are intended for the birthing person to attend alone.

The need for support and the challenges of parenthood apply to all parents. Every parent will have unique parenting and interpersonal skills that will impact their infant's development, supporting the child to thrive, mature and develop emotional wellbeing (Greenfield & Darwin, 2021).

SUMMARY

Parents require knowledge and support to experience healthy pregnancies and build strong foundations for the future wellbeing of themselves and their infants. The importance of good mental health cannot be overstated because of the impact it has on families and society and, of course, on the life of the parent themselves. Many parents may use the internet to find the information they require in the perinatal period, but it often doesn't provide them with reliable, evidence-based sources. This is why the work of practitioners, who are best trained and placed to support parents in the perinatal period, is of such significance and value.

There are many risk factors for, and presentations of, mental health conditions during pregnancy. It is not possible to prevent or solve all of them, but if you, as a practitioner, can develop the knowledge, skills and resources to be able to identify them, you can help to ensure that parents feel well supported and equipped with possible approaches to managing challenging situations and experiences.

CHAPTER 2

Perinatal Mental Health – Family and Society

IMPACTS OF PERINATAL MENTAL HEALTH CONDITIONS

The significant impacts that perinatal mental health conditions can have on family wellbeing mean that early diagnosis, treatment and support are critical to achieving positive long-term outcomes (Aarestrup *et al.*, 2020; Howard, Poit & Stein, 2014). Anxiety and depression can pass down from generation to generation, and if a parent's depression is left untreated, it can have adverse consequences for their child. Perinatal mental health conditions can affect:

- mothers
- fathers
- infants and children
- adolescents
- grandparents
- society.

Impacts on mothers

The impact of depression on mothers can be significant. Sadly, suicide is the fifth most common cause of women's deaths during pregnancy and shortly following the birth of the infant (MBRACCE-UK, 2020).

Nearly half of the women who died by suicide were known to psychiatric services and half of that number had been admitted to a psychiatric unit following childbirth (MBRACCE-UK, 2020). Social services were involved in the lives of 17% of women who died (Khalifa *et al.*, 2016). In high-income countries, a higher proportion of men than women lose their lives to suicide, while in low-income countries suicide rates are higher for women (Chin *et al.*, 2022; WHO, 2023). Currently, there are no specific statistics recording the number of fathers who have died by suicide.

NHS England offer some practice tips for ways to include the whole family in the mother's mental health care (see box).[1] The following box is from the guide *Involving and supporting partners and other family members in specialist perinatal mental health services: Good practice guide* (Darwin *et al.*, 2021).

Practical tips to help the practitioner

Ask open questions to discover who is included in the family system and who is important to the mother without making assumptions. Stay curious.

- Who is in the family system, and how are these relationships experienced?
- Who may give consent for the information that she has shared?
- Who may she want to be invited into assessment or treatment sessions, or to be involved in aspects of her care?
- Who would she want to be told about her involvement in the service and who would she not want to be told?
- Who is she close to? Is there anyone she has a more difficult relationship with?
- Who does she turn to for support? Who does she feel is not supportive?

1 See www.england.nhs.uk/mental-health/perinatal/perinatal-mental-health-resources for these and more resources and practice tips for perinatal mental health from NHS England.

What are the culture, beliefs and values within the family system? These will affect the approaches needed to foster engagement.

- How is the role of men/fathers viewed? Are fathers expected to be involved in childcare, or would this be unusual? Be sensitive to different cultural, ethnic and religious influences.
- How are mental health disorders and services viewed? Is she worried about the views of other family members, and does she plan to keep her involvement with the service hidden from them?
- Who has similar/different values and beliefs to the mother?

Which other services or groups may be important?

- Has she received support from other health or mental health care providers, third sector organisations, religious or community groups? What did she find helpful?
- Does she have other networks that are important to her (for example work or social networks)?'

Impacts on fathers

Dr Blaithin O'Dea, Child Psychologist in the Perinatal Community Team, Southern Health NHS Foundation Trust, describes some of the potential mental health problems for fathers:

> Fathers are often identified by mothers and indeed professionals as the 'support system' for the mother. Whilst this is an obvious role for them, it means they are expected to become the one taking care of the mother, the doer, the strong one, the 'container'. This is a challenging task for anyone and, for new dads who are sleep deprived, adjusting to huge changes and likely worried about their partners, it may be an overwhelming task. This is compounded by the fact that supportive

> contacts from midwives and health visitors after a baby is born are almost entirely focused on the wellbeing of mum and baby. The expectation that dad will provide support and stability can create intense pressure, uncertainty and feelings of inadequacy for fathers which are justified, valid and need support. (O'Dea, quoted in Williams, 2020)

Studies show that a father's depression may adversely affect family functioning, cause conflict between partners and induce depressive symptoms in the mother (Ramchandani *et al.*, 2008). More recent research suggests that one in 20 new fathers experience depression in the weeks following the birth of their infant (Hambidge *et al.*, 2021). If a mother is depressed, it can have a significant impact on a father, and it may exacerbate problems with their mental health (Kim & Swain, 2007; Kiviruusu *et al.*, 2020; Wee *et al.*, 2011).

The effects that a traumatic birth may have on a mother are well documented (Ertan *et al.*, 2021; Reed, Sharman & Inglis, 2017), but the impact of witnessing a traumatic birth on fathers has been largely under-reported. A father may have watched their partner receiving urgent surgical interventions or experienced their partner's or child's life being at risk. A recent study suggests that the speed and unexpected turn of events in some traumatic births paralysed some fathers who were excluded while medical teams tried to save lives. Fathers reported feeling powerless to intervene and unable to offer help except to support the mother (Etheridge & Slade, 2017).

Self-harm and suicidal ideation can affect new fathers. A significant proportion of men have admitted to experiencing suicidal or self-harm thoughts during the early years of parenting. Studies have shown that approximately 1 in 25 fathers of young children may experience these thoughts. (Fogarty *et al.*, 2024). This self-harm may often be interpreted as an accident. If fathers do not receive treatment and support for depressive symptoms during the perinatal period, it can impact the whole family, often resulting in fathers using negative coping skills, avoiding emotionally challenging situations and feeling angry. Unfortunately, very few fathers are asked about their mental health or are individually assessed after becoming a parent despite experiencing physiological and psychological changes in the perinatal period. In recent research, it has been found that fathers' testosterone, cortisol and oestrogen levels lower at this time as a natural adaptation to parenthood (Edelstein *et al.*, 2014; Saxbe *et al.*, 2017). This natural hormonal adjustment is believed to facilitate a greater focus on the care and nurturing of the infant and to facilitate greater bonding with the infant.

There is currently an emphasis on assessing and or screening fathers' mental health during the perinatal period. Historically, assessment tools, which include the Edinburgh Postnatal Depression Scale (EPDS), have been designed for mothers, and it is the mother who is requested to answer the ten questions during the antenatal and postnatal periods, in order to determine how she is feeling. The lack of a similar assessment for men means that the mental health of the father can easily be missed, and as a result they will slip under the radar with their wellbeing not being considered. The EPDS has been validated for fathers by Matthey *et al.* (2001).

Men may show symptoms of distress in a different way to women. The co-author of this book, Mark Williams, shared the following suggested prompts to help partners feel more comfortable talking about distress:

- 'This can be such a stressful time – you're concerned both for your partner and your baby and there are lots of unknowns.'
- 'Some partners can end up feeling guilty or blaming themselves. For example, they have had thoughts like, "Why is she depressed? Is it me? Doesn't she want the baby?"'
- 'Around half of partners feel depressed, anxious or very stressed themselves when their partner is unwell. You could be struggling as well and we need to think about you, too.'

- 'Watching a difficult birth can be very upsetting. Often, people can feel panicky or out of control.'[2]

Impacts on infants and children

An infant is totally dependent on its parent(s) and is highly motivated to connect with them. For infants' emotional development to be healthy, certain needs must be met. These needs include love, attention, warmth, good nutrition, sufficient sleep, sensory stimulation and feeling secure.

Young babies cannot communicate their needs verbally and parents may find it challenging to interpret and respond to their child's requirements. Of course, not all parent and infant relationships will be consistently positive. However, learning that challenges in interacting can be resolved helps the parent to build strong bonds with the infant.

During pregnancy

As foetuses are sensitive to adverse maternal environments, a mother's mental health is an important consideration throughout pregnancy. The environment in the womb is important, as, excluding pregnancies where there are greater complications, the healthier the environment, the healthier the newborn infant. Factors promoting infant health include mothers having a nutritious diet, getting sufficient sleep, and avoiding alcohol and drugs.

There is still much to be learned about the effects of stress or distress during pregnancy. Stress can occur at any time and in different forms, from relationship difficulties to experiencing natural disasters. Such sources of stress may have permanent effects on the development of the foetus (Glover *et al.*, 2018). Hormones play an important role in a mother's behaviour during pregnancy. If a mother is subjected to stressful situations, she will produce higher amounts of cortisol or

2 Reproduced from: https://www.england.nhs.uk/mental-health/perinatal/perinatal-mental-health-resources/involving-and-supporting-partners-and-other-family-members-in-specialist-perinatal-mental-health-services-good-practice-guide/idea-4-partners-and-other-family-members-own-mental-health-needs/

stress hormone. This crosses the placenta, giving the unborn infant elevated levels of cortisol in their bloodstream. Although research determining how maternal stress affects in utero brain development is ongoing (Nath *et al.*, 2017), studies have found that an overload of stress results in what is now termed 'toxic stress' (Stidham Hall *et al.*, 2019).

Evidence from many studies has associated toxic stress in mothers during pregnancy with heightened cortisol levels in infants (Babenkeo, Kovalchuk & Metz, 2015; Glover, 2014; Gross *et al.*, 2016). This is associated with outcomes including the premature birth of the infant, the infant having a lower birth weight than was expected, and the infant's immune system being altered. Studies have found that infants affected by toxic stress may have a more difficult temperament than was anticipated, often finding it difficult to settle and sleeping poorly. It is important to note that the causes of many conditions are complex. While some studies suggest children affected by toxic stress may present with behavioural problems, conduct disorders or neurodivergent conditions (Erhuma, 2021) and be more likely to have attention deficit disorder (ADD), autism and poor cognitive development (Beversdorf *et al.*, 2019; Grizenko *et al.*, 2012; Reissland *et al.*, 2015) there is no single gene that causes ADHD or depression, but many variations, each of which makes a small contribution and interacts with environmental factors, starting in the womb.

Support around stress should be non-stigmatising – be aware that there are unhelpful narratives that blame parents for conditions that their child might have. A neuro-affirmative approach looks to ensure that neurodivergence is not framed as a defect, but rather part of human neurodiversity (O'Dell *et al.*, 2025).

During the postnatal period

The mental health of either or both parents can have an effect on an infant or child's cognitive development, reciprocity and social attachment. Infant mental health is the emotional wellbeing of an infant during the period when the brain is growing rapidly, from birth to three years of age. Promoting healthy brain maturation from the start of the perinatal period supports the social, emotional and cognitive development of infants.

After birth, the most important things that infants need during any stage in their development is connection with their parents, in the form of presence and affection. Infants thrive on warmth, kind-heartedness and love. In the first month, infants are fascinated by their parents' faces. A month later, more complex patterns of behaviour start to form, with infants becoming more visually alert and aware of their parents' expressions. This is evidenced by infants' reactions when their parents smile, gaze and make cooing voices at them. Infants gradually become more attuned to their parents, slowly building confidence and learning to socialise by conversing, playing games and becoming comfortable with others. These behaviours do not need to be learnt as they are innate and prepare a parent and their infant for their future interactions (Trevarthen & Aitken, 2001).

For parents who are anxious or depressed, meeting their child's needs can be a challenge. A parent can be struggling with their own emotions and find it difficult to feel joy; they may unintentionally express how they feel, and the infant recognises this. A lack of emotion from a parent can make an infant feel insecure and vulnerable. A parent may be preoccupied by intrusive negative thoughts of not feeling good enough because they cannot get their infant to settle or they feel that the infant would rather be with anyone else than them. Depressive symptoms can make parents lethargic and exhausted, compounded if they are experiencing sleepless nights with their infant. This can make domestic chores demanding, leaving parents with little energy to cope with the pressures of caring for the infant.

Support strategies for infants and children

To help a parent manage their infant, a practitioner must ensure that the parent receives appropriate support for any difficulties and treatment for any mental health condition they may be experiencing.

During the perinatal period, practitioners can share practical tips to encourage parents to bond and care for their infant, such as suggesting that parents create a daily opportunity to spend quality time with their infant. Parents can also be supported to understand and acknowledge why their infant may be distressed, and to learn to reassure their infant that they will be attended to as soon as possible. Showing parents that cuddling and hugging their infant can enable the infant to learn that the parent understands how they are feeling, though not necessarily why, may be reassuring for parents too. Infants' wellbeing will be promoted by encouraging parents to respond to the infant's crying, sadness or frustration with loving gestures, and simple playful gestures of blowing raspberries, singing or dancing. These interactions can support bonding, develop the infant's cognitive behaviour, give them emotional strength, and help them to develop the capacity to know that they are safe and secure.

Impacts on adolescents

Some adolescents will have a parent who has experienced an episode of a treatable mental health condition, while others will have a parent with a long-term mental health condition, such as drug and or alcohol misuse. A smaller proportion of adolescents live with a parent who has a severe mental illness, such as bipolar disorder or psychosis.

Many children will not be affected by their parent's disorder. However, studies researching the impact of a parent's perinatal mental disorder show that the risk of a 16-year-old having depression when their mother had antenatal depression was almost five times greater than for those mothers who had not experienced antenatal depression (Pawlby *et al.*, 2009; Plant *et al.*, 2015). If therapeutic interventions for parents are not accessed, it can have repercussions for children as they develop. This may lead to disorders including depression or substance misuse, and an elevated risk of suicidal ideation or self-harming behaviours.

Adolescents whose parents are expecting another baby or have a young infant may not understand what is happening to a parent who may be depressed or anxious whilst pregnant or when their sibling is newly born. An adolescent may feel unable to talk with their parent about their emotions, sometimes compounded by poor interactions due to their parent's depression or anxiety, and they may feel alienated or isolated from them. Some parents may try to protect their child from their illness refusing to discuss it or attempting to keep it secret by disguising how they really feel. This may cause unreasonable actions because the adolescent can only internalise their grief, sometimes making them angry at the disconnection with their parent. Often, they might find it difficult to control their reactions or emotions, and their emotional response may be excessive, such as becoming increasingly obstinate or argumentative, making unreasonable demands or being verbally abusive. This can sometimes influence their behaviour causing direct or unintentional harm to others.

If a mother with a mental health condition is admitted to a mother and baby unit, there may be expectations that their adolescent child will take on additional domestic duties. As a result, they may miss days at school, which will have an impact on their education. If the mother is not admitted, then the adolescent may need to assume a caring role for their parent and their infant sibling.

Adolescents are more likely to able to cope if they understand their parent's mental health condition. However, this can cause problems as they may be aware of what is happening but feel as if they are not trusted or mature enough to deal with their parent's condition. Some evidence suggests that with this feeling of distrust, adolescents are more likely to internalise how they feel and are more likely to exhibit behavioural problems (Gladstone *et al.*, 2011).

Adolescents may also feel guilty because they think that their parent's illness is their fault. Despite support being in place, adolescents may still have feelings of anxiety, shame and distress due to their parent's illness or behaviours. They may hide these fears and be preoccupied by feelings that they too will suffer from a similar illness. Sometimes, because of the insensitivity of their peers and the impact of stigma, adolescents may be bullied and teased. Many adolescents suffer from low self-esteem and believe that their problems are unique, and they often feel that any worries they have are dismissed by others as they are not deemed important enough. There is a risk that adolescents whose parents are experiencing issues with perinatal mental health may become withdrawn because of their overwhelming responsibilities and the challenge of trusting anyone to talk to about their parent's illness.

Not only do adolescents have to cope with an ill parent, they also have to manage their own transition from child to adult. During this developmental period, the desire to develop a new identity and independence can lead to experimentation and risk-taking, therefore it is important for practitioners to understand how taking on the caring responsibilities of the parent can impact on their own mental health (Simpson, 2020).

Support strategies for adolescents

Understanding their parent's illness or disorder can help adolescents to learn coping strategies. Practitioners can provide adolescents with resources that explain what is happening to their parent. Adolescents need to understand that they cannot change the way their parent behaves, but they can have compassion for themselves and seek support from family and friends. They can be referred to support groups within their area and access services dedicated to helping children, such as Childline, which offers phone and online support.

Despite the challenges they experience, with the right understanding and recognition, adolescents can learn to view their experiences as a part of post-traumatic growth, which may enable them to flourish and gain a greater understanding and appreciation of mental health conditions. Practitioners can discuss the positive personal qualities the teenager has gained from their life experiences and how that will help them to flourish with their future life choices.

Impacts on grandparents

Grandparents are often important sources of support and stability in the face of major family upheavals, such as the breakdown of relationships, moving house or health issues. Just as the birth of an infant brings significant changes to the identities, responsibilities and relationships of new parents, it can also significantly affect grandparents' lives.

New parents can feel exhausted, vulnerable and desperate for practical support. They can be disappointed when their expectations of parenting are not met, and they need to be able to verbalise how they feel. Grandparents can help the parents to navigate the early days of parenthood, whilst also respecting their autonomy. They can offer practical support by providing childcare, preparing meals and helping with household tasks to enable the new mother to rest and recuperate. They can suggest techniques to help mothers to breastfeed their infant, whilst at the same time offering a supportive listening ear and encouraging them to persevere, particularly if the mother is facing difficulties, both emotionally and practically (Honikman, 2022; Scelza & Hinde, 2019).

However, grandparents' ideas about their role can be confusing; some grandparents may feel shut out of their grandchildren's lives or feel overly responsible for them. Grandparents may be able to buffer some stress associated with the transition to parenthood, but they can also become a source of stress for expectant couples by offering advice that conflicts with guidance from practitioners.

Support strategies for relationships with grandparents

Grandparents are an important resource who can, in some cases, reduce stress and ease parents' transitions during the perinatal period. It is important that new parents, who are simultaneously grappling with their own recoveries and perhaps the fragile health of their infant, are aware that social support is key to coping with these challenges. This can be provided by strengthening the family system to widen the circle of support and by building and sustaining a sense of belonging within a community. Grandparents are often just needed to be there, not necessarily to become overly involved, but to reassure and support younger generations.

Impacts on society

As well as impacting health and wellbeing, perinatal mental health conditions can affect the resources and finances available within societies. If society addressed the unmet needs of maternal mental health, it would have an economic benefit of £490 million over ten years: a significant proportion of this (over 75%) relates to impacts on the child (Bauer *et al.*, 2022).

Perinatal mental health is everybody's responsibility. Changing attitudes within society have made discussions around perinatal mental health more acceptable and mainstream, increasing our understanding of the challenges and needs that parents experience. We must continue to listen to parents to learn how to create a society that supports them effectively. This will make it easier to confront barriers to improving perinatal mental health and to make the most of opportunities to promote family wellbeing. Education and prevention within society is the key, taking every opportunity to talk about the cause and effect of perinatal mental health can help parents. Practitioners can support parents by providing them with evidence-based knowledge about becoming a parent, considering the many privileges and pitfalls they may experience, so that they are prepared for any eventualities that may occur.

Support strategies

It is important for practitioners to acknowledge that, often, it is the wider family and society who are concerned about the health and wellbeing of a parent who is displaying symptoms of a perinatal mental health condition. A parent may think their feelings are temporary while they attempt to find a life, work and baby balance, but their family and friends believe that the parent's suffering is more serious. Taking the concerns of a parent's family and friends seriously is vital as no parent should suffer unnecessarily from any mental health condition.

Practitioners should use their skills and knowledge to contribute to equipping future generations to be mentally resilient, robust and well. Providing this foundation will enable parents to enjoy parenthood as fully as possible and help infants to achieve the best possible start in life.

IMPACTS OF SOCIETAL ATTITUDES ON MENTAL HEALTH

Stigma is often viewed as negative, and very often unfair, beliefs that a family, society or group of people have about something or somebody. When it comes to perinatal mental health, stigma and systemic barriers can be directed towards both the mother's and the father's condition. This feeling of being stigmatised can result in embarrassment and shame and is often coupled with a reluctance to share their emotions with anyone. Sometimes, this makes it difficult for even the parent to admit to themselves how they are feeling.

There are many societal misconceptions about parenthood. Parents may feel their abilities are being judged and they should conform to certain cultural norms. The parent may not be able to admit how they feel as they expect to be judged and labelled as an unfit parent, and as a consequence their infant will be removed from their care.

Taking prescribed antidepressants or antipsychotic medication can be difficult for the parent to reconcile, and sometimes the need for vital medication is criticised by others as being unnecessary. However, the same argument would not happen if the parent was taking an antibiotic, and yet the drugs are equally important.

Even in our considered age, for the uninitiated, it is not just the silent opinions that matter, but the vocal attitudes which deem anyone suffering from anxiety as 'weak' or 'attention-seeking' and needing to 'snap out of it', whilst depression may be viewed as 'incompetence' or a personal weakness that can be overcome by willpower.

In some societies there are cultural taboos about perinatal mental health. If the parent feels they will be judged by their friends, family and members of their community, there may be a reluctance to even discuss how they are feeling, with a tendency to remain silent and uncommunicative about their condition. Sometimes, this can be misinterpreted by health practitioners as the mother's refusal to engage, however, the mother feels she is keeping safe and protecting her family members, who by association, may also be stigmatised.

It is important to be culturally sensitive and to understand that social inequities and experiences with racism and discrimination can compound the stigma faced and felt by racial and ethnic minorities, and as a result their mental health may deteriorate.

Facing this insidious torrent of abusive behaviour can be destabilising, with consequences for the deterioration of the parents' mental health. Therefore, it is important that the family are aware of the damaging misinterpretations of mental health. With their knowledge and support, the family are able to help the parent to have the confidence to seek medical help and accept the therapies offered, whilst assuring the parent that they are caring, there is little chance of their infant being taken into care, and they will be there for them throughout their recovery.

SUMMARY

For a person to develop and maintain the best possible mental health, the rudiments of their wellbeing must be recognised throughout the lifespan. In the context of perinatal mental health, the chicken-and-egg scenario applies to considerations about whether it is wisest to focus on the healthy lifestyle of mothers, fathers, foetuses or infants. Their wellbeing is profoundly inter-related, and to achieve positive outcomes all family members must be supported both antenatally and postnatally. The infant requires a healthy environment to secure the optimum development of their neurological and physical systems. Beginning the journey of supporting parents to create a nurturing environment in the pre-conception stages ensures that both mothers and fathers can access healthy lifestyle choices from the outset. Providing ongoing whole-family support and, when necessary, effective mental health interventions will build on these foundations.

During the perinatal period, practitioners can make a significant difference to the mental health of a parent. Their skills and knowledge can help to effectively support parents in what can be a challenging time, enabling them to manage and thrive.

USEFUL RESOURCES

Support for children and adolescents

Action for Children: www.actionforchildren.org.uk

Barnardo's: www.barnardos.org.uk

Childline: www.childline.org.uk

The Children's Society: www.childrenssociety.org.uk

YoungMinds: www.youngminds.org.uk

NSPCC: www.nspcc.org.uk

Support for grandparents

Family Lives offers advice and information for grandparents, including tips on supporting your grandchildren with childcare and health, and information about kinship care if your grandchildren come to live with you: www.familylives.org.uk/advice/your-family/grandparents

CHAPTER-SPECIFIC WORKSHEETS FOR PRACTITIONERS (SEE APPENDIX)

Worksheet 1: Pregnancy

Worksheet 2: Supporting fathers in the antenatal period

Worksheet 3: The perinatal period

Worksheet 4: Thinking about older children

Worksheet 5: Lifestyle choices in the perinatal period

Worksheet 6: Interactions between mood and lifestyle

CHAPTER 3

Risk and Protective Factors for Perinatal Mental Health

Many factors during both the antenatal and postnatal periods can pose risks to parents' mental health. Risk factors around the time of labour and delivery may include a difficult labour, a traumatic delivery or complications with the health of the infant. Postnatally, practitioners need a thorough awareness of the risks to mental health throughout the perinatal period because forming a holistic picture of parents' mental wellbeing depends on understanding the risk factors parents have been exposed to.

This chapter outlines some of the most significant risk and protective factors that can affect family wellbeing during the perinatal period and provides suggestions for how practitioners can most effectively support parents at this important time.

RISK FACTORS

Risk factors that can have a significant influence on parents' mental health include economic pressures, bereavement, relationship difficulties, war trauma, and exposure to environmental disasters and public health crises (such as the Covid-19 pandemic).

Bereavement

The death or illness of a supportive figure, for example, the mother's mother, can significantly affect parents' mental health (Persson & Rossin-Slater, 2018). Stress and anxiety caused by this challenging experience can be amplified if it occurs around the time of the birth, or the mother does not receive adequate or timely support (Cacciatore, Killian & Harper, 2016). Although it is too soon for evidence to establish the impact of the pandemic on mothers who had to give birth without their usual support network, anecdotal evidence from practitioners suggests that these mothers may need extra interventions and support during the coming years.

Perinatal loss

As one in five pregnancies ends in miscarriage it is important to consider the effect that this will have on both parents' mental health. Some mothers, partners or other family members may have experienced pregnancy loss or the death of a baby before or during the current episode of care. Regardless of gestation, age, or reason, such losses can exacerbate pre-existing mental health disorders or precipitate new mental health difficulties.

> Any parent who has experienced perinatal loss is at increased risk of depression, anxiety disorders, including tokophobia (extreme fear of childbirth) and birth-related trauma. Grief itself should not be pathologised, and it is important to ensure that mental health needs and symptoms are not mistakenly attributed to grief (NHS England, n.d.).

Trauma

War trauma

Parents who have experienced war, civil unrest, economic disaster and/or poverty, and who may have been forced to flee to a safer environment, have their own challenges. Disenfranchised from familiar lifestyles, parents who are refugees may have to adapt to different living standards and cultural values. Parents with high levels of resilience may cope effectively with such trauma and adjustment, but for vulnerable pregnant women and infants, these experiences are risk factors for developing mental health issues in the perinatal period.

Exposure to traumatic experiences can have serious psychological outcomes. Post-traumatic stress disorder (PTSD) after experiencing conflict is common. A study by Musisi and Kinyanda (2020) demonstrated how the trauma suffered in conflict and post-conflict settings in Africa surfaced in the population, with increased numbers of people suffering from anxiety and depression. Escalating wars and the damage they cause in places such as Syria, Afghanistan and Ukraine, are widely reported by the media, revealing the horrors inflicted on civilians. It is unsurprising that this exposure to war trauma has serious negative effects on maternal wellbeing; studies relating to conflict exposure have found that mothers' distress and depression is often associated with their children's distress (Qouta *et al.*, 2005).

Environmental disasters

The unpredictable weather associated with climate change has consequences for society and mental health. Wildfires in the USA, Australia and Europe have had catastrophic outcomes for families, causing terror about possible injury, death and damage to properties. The impact of this on perinatal mental health can be severe (Amjad *et al.*, 2021; Verstraeten *et al.*, 2021). Overwhelming anxiety and sleep disturbances appear to be the most common responses before, during and after wildfires.

Media reports also highlight rising water levels and the risk of many countries being submerged in the future, while villages and towns in the UK have been subjected to unprecedented floods that have destroyed homes and businesses. Natural disasters can create a significant psychological legacy; earthquake survivors were found to be at higher risk of experiencing depression 37 years after surviving an earthquake (Gao *et al.*, 2019).

The Covid-19 pandemic

Wei *et al.* (2021) found that Covid-19 infection during pregnancy was associated with risks of pre-eclampsia, stillbirth, preterm birth and neonatal intensive care admission. There has also been an increase in mental health illnesses and disorders and family disruption, and a decrease in mother-to-child attachment (Singh *et al.*, 2020). It is clear that the pandemic took a toll on children and families, and the resulting increased pressure on family services meant that some families' needs were not met. The Children's Commissioner for England (2024) highlighted a concerning trend in the mental health of children who are already engaged with support services and suggested that existing support systems were not adequate to address the growing needs of children. During the pandemic, there were instances where some parents experienced many risk factors for perinatal mental health issues, including loneliness, bereavement and limited access to support and services. These families must now be effectively supported to limit the transmission of poor mental health across generations.

During lockdowns, there was an increase in the number of pregnant women presenting with mental distress at their first antenatal appointment (Campos-Garzón *et al.*, 2021). However, initially there appeared to be no change in referral rates to secondary care services. Worryingly, there was a decrease in the number of women reporting incidents of domestic violence, highlighting the need to ask pregnant women about domestic violence rather than assuming that they will reveal this independently.

Insomnia triggered by stressful or traumatic events was widely reported during the pandemic (Wang *et al.*, 2021). Adequate good-quality sleep is needed for parents to maintain good perinatal mental health. Sleep problems can arise if a parent is suffering from anxiety and spends their time ruminating. This can make it difficult to adjust to a regular bedtime routine; as a result, the mind cannot adequately deal with painful experiences and is left with negative emotions (Robillard *et al.*, 2020).

The Covid-19 pandemic has highlighted how vulnerable to mental illness parents can be when they are isolated from their extended families, friends and communities, and when they experience stress due to the loss of employment and rising prices.

Domestic abuse

Studies indicate that over 30% of domestic abuse incidents against women start whilst the woman is pregnant. Approximately 15% of women have reported a violent episode during their pregnancy, while over half have admitted to violent experiences (Alhusen *et al.*, 2015).

Domestic abuse can take many forms. Domestic abuse isn't always physical; where this is the case, it is often described as an incident, or a pattern of incidents, whereby the partner is persistently emotionally abused by being threatened, humiliated and violated. This is often known as 'coercive control'.

The partner can also be subjected to physical, sexual abuse or intimate partner violence. The perpetrator is usually male but can also be female. One in seven women and one in twenty-five men have been injured by an intimate partner (NCADV, 2024). Domestic violence is more likely to intensify during pregnancy. Challenges during pregnancy, such as jealousy from the shift in attention towards the pregnancy, or stress from an unplanned pregnancy and its potential financial strain, can contribute to an environment where existing abuse escalates.

Reports of domestic violence rose significantly during the Covid-19 lockdowns (Usta, Murr & El-Jarrah, 2021).

Interventions for domestic abuse

Building a trusting and respectful discussion with the parent can enable practitioners to challenge and discuss abusive or controlling attitudes. It is important to remember that these might be fostered by an undetected depressive illness or feelings of anxiety. Openly talking about how a parent is really feeling may help to reveal relevant information about their abusive relationship and its impact on their family and themselves.

Both physical violence and coercive control are criminal offences and can be reported to the police. In 2015, the offence of controlling or coercive behaviour (CCB) came into force through Section 76 of the Serious Crime Act. The police may give the abuser a warning or they may arrest them for a criminal offence. If the police have enough evidence, they will refer the matter to the Crown Prosecution Service.

With specific reference to abuse against women, interventions can be either gender-intentional, which include working mainly with women, or gender-transformative, where the environment in which women live is altered by working with both the systems and the men in the women's lives. Working with men in a gender-transformative way by encouraging them to become more involved with their infant and the mother, and supporting gender equity, have been found to be successful approaches to reducing domestic violence. Many programmes aim to reduce domestic violence by having one-stop centres to identify abuse at every point of contact, such as through obstetric, gynaecological and maternal health services. This includes fathers, brothers and uncles. Studies suggest that education and economic security are also significant (Dong, Xue & Yaqin, 2021).

Safeguarding

Safeguarding means the protection of parents, their children or family from harm, abuse, exploitation, maltreatment and neglect. It is of paramount importance, as it ensures the wellbeing of the parents and the family throughout the perinatal period. Through recognising and addressing any risk factors, dismantling the barriers of detection and ensuring there is access to appropriate services, interventions can be implemented early and be more effective.

The signs that the consideration of safeguarding is essential are, the indication of a suicide risk, recent thoughts or acts of violent self-harm, a significant deterioration in the parent's mental state, persistent expressions of uselessness or incompetence as a parent or diminishing attachment with the infant.

It is the core responsibility of all healthcare practitioners, as outlined in the Mental Health Act 2007, to consider the wellbeing of the family. This act is designed to ensure that those with a serious mental health disorder, which may threaten their safety and the wellbeing or the safety of others, or where it is necessary to prevent them from harming themselves or others, are able to be treated irrespective of their consent. It is often the family who are first aware of the worsening of the parent's mental state, and it is important that they are able to discuss their concerns openly and freely without any prejudice. It is equally important to ensure that any planned interventions or options are explored with the parent and the family, as these decisions will affect the family as a whole.

PROTECTIVE FACTORS

In the postnatal period, protective factors that can promote bonding and reduce the risk of perinatal mental health issues include skin-to-skin contact and breastfeeding.

Skin-to-skin contact

This is sometimes offered directly after the birth of the infant and is encouraged as the infant develops. The infant is laid on their tummy and placed directly onto the parent's bare chest. This process promotes bonding between the parent and the infant, enabling the infant to connect to their parent by feeling safe and protected. It can be particularly important when a family has experienced trauma and may need support to bond with their child.

Skin-to-skin contact also has advantages for breastfeeding as it can make the nursing process easier. Pre-term and low birthweight infants who had skin-to-skin initiated breastfeeding almost three days earlier than mothers who received conventional care of the incubator method (Mekonnen, Yehualashet & Bayleyegn, 2019).

Gitau *et al.* (cited in Ionio, Ciuffo & Landoni, 2021) found that just 20 minutes of maternal skin-to-skin contact caused a significant and consistent reduction in cortisol levels. Studies have also shown that a delay in skin-to-skin contact contributed to a decline in maternal responses to infants' cues, sometimes lasting as long as a year. It has been suggested it can lower the risk of postpartum depression (Cooijmans *et al.*, 2017). The benefits relate to fathers too; one study reports that in cases where infants were born by caesarean section, fathers who practised skin-to-skin contact with their infant appeared to have lower scores of anxiety and depression, and felt they achieved the role of being a father because their instincts were triggered through consistent skin-to-skin time (Huang *et al.*, 2019).

Breastfeeding

An overwhelming amount of research indicates that breastfeeding is best for the infant, and significant information suggests that breastfeeding mothers who have strong social support from their partner are more likely to initiate and continue the process (Brown & Davies, 2014). Studies have shown that breastfeeding may have a preventative effect on maternal mental health conditions developing.

A study by Borra, Iacovou and Sevilla (2015) showed that mothers who planned to and went on to breastfeed were about 50% less likely to become depressed than mothers who had not planned to, and who did not, breastfeed. However, it's important to recognise that some mothers understand the benefits of breastfeeding and would like to continue but, because of their mental state or physical reasons, feel unable to do so. The same study showed that mothers who planned to breastfeed but were unable to, were over twice as likely to become depressed. Mothers may need support in dealing with feelings of shame or failure. The study also found that the relationship between breastfeeding and depression was most pronounced when babies were eight weeks old but was much smaller when babies were eight months or older.

If parents receive sufficient information from the practitioner about the processes of breastfeeding, they will feel more informed and confident (Brown, Raynor & Lee, 2011). This is true in many cultures, as mothers who have the support of their partner report feeling more capable and competent when making breastfeeding decisions (Mannion *et al.*, 2013). There may, however, be cultural contexts where paternal involvement in breastfeeding is limited. Fathers may also benefit from the opportunity to read about or talk to fathers who have become more confident about their ability to support the mother and have been able to overcome any embarrassment or uncertainty in relation to breastfeeding. This can only enhance both parents' confidence and self-esteem, which in turn will help to minimise any feelings of anxiety or inadequacy.

One of the largest surveys conducted in the UK about fathers' thoughts on breastfeeding found that that 92% of the fathers who responded said they required more information in order to be able to better support their partner's breastfeeding (Howl, 2019).

The influence of grandparents can make a real difference to the success of breastfeeding mothers. Some who may have experienced, and overcome difficulties, for example about infants latching onto the breast or the timing of feeds, are able to pass on that knowledge and skill to support both mothers and fathers. The grandparent may be familiar with the importance of persisting with breastfeeding and encourage the mother not to give up. The grandmother may also have recollections about how her own perinatal emotions prevented her from enjoying breastfeeding and therefore be able to empathise with her daughter's feelings. However, it is also important to recognise when the mother is struggling and not to make judgements on her inability to, or desire not to, breastfeed as a result of the mother's low mood state.

Should the father or partner have to work, a grandparent can offer practical help around the house with the domestic chores or shopping, thus allowing the mother to have the much-needed rest she requires to breastfeed her baby. Although it is easy to give advice, many grandparents are well placed to know and understand when it is better to listen to the concerns and to continue to encourage the mother and father in whatever they decide to do, as it will always be the best decision.

Overall wellbeing

Evidence suggests that parents who access their communities through social support have described positive outcomes for their health and wellbeing (Coates, Davis & Campbell, 2017). These outcomes include improved quality of life, positive emotional experiences, and promotion of their self-care. As in other studies, the act of belonging to a community or peer support group and the parent knowing and feeling that they have an important role to play has a significant impact on reducing anxiety or feelings of loneliness. Practitioners can facilitate this and help families to secure a more productive and less stressful future. However, there are limitations to a practitioner's role, and it is important to recognise when help should be sought to further support parents. A background knowledge of perinatal mental health services, appropriate support groups and interventions that practitioners are confident conducting, all help with the process.

MALADAPTIVE COPING MECHANISMS

Some parents may self-medicate to try and alleviate feelings of distress rather than seeking medical help. This may be because they fear possible stigma of admitting that they are 'unable to cope' and the potential consequences if they admit to their feelings. There are several types of self-medication including:

- substance misuse
- use of caffeine
- smoking
- alcohol misuse
- gambling.

Substance misuse

Substance misuse is often associated with the symptoms of anxiety or depression. The problem is that it is a vicious cycle, because taking drugs to alleviate these symptoms is more likely to intensify anxiety or depression. Initially, drugs may minimise or make the symptoms more bearable, and this respite can encourage greater drug use. The elation felt from the effects is only temporary, and seeking the same effect can lead to increased abuse and physical problems, as well as addiction, and the worsening of mood disorders.

Cocaine is also growing in popularity as a recreational drug (Home Office, 2019). It constricts blood vessels and can have poor results for the baby in utero: the placenta may separate; the brain, organs and limbs may not develop properly; and more severe usage may cause a stillbirth or miscarriage. Benzodiazepines, which include Valium, Temazepam, Librium and Nitrazepam can be purchased as 'street drugs' (McAuley *et al.*, 2025). These drugs were originally developed as muscle relaxants but because of their mood-altering effects, they were prescribed for stress. They should be used in caution during pregnancy as they can cause withdrawal symptoms in the infant, and there is some evidence to suggest there is a slightly increased risk of cleft palate, although the risk is relatively small (Teng & Steinbacher, 2013).

Warning signs of substance abuse may include:

- becoming dependent on the amount of substance it takes to 'feel better'
- fear of not being able to access the substance and the stress this causes
- needing to be secretive about the amount of the substance consumed.

Substance abuse can result in parents being dishonest with themselves and others. Parents may also justify their reasons for taking substances by suggesting they are primarily medicating to prevent or relieve the feelings of stress. The way in which substances interfere with lifestyles is often insidious, and it is usually family members who notice the deterioration in behaviours and moods. Encouraging parents to seek help as soon as the 'condition' presents can help to halt any further decline in both the physical and mental health of the parent. There are specialist services that are familiar with drug and alcohol misuse, and they should be contacted to ensure the mother, and the family, get the help they deserve.

The period after the birth is a critical time as some surveys imply that there is a high prevalence of alcohol and illicit drug use in new mothers, suggesting that some postnatal depressions are related to substance use. (Chapman & Wu, 2013). Mothers who are already depressed may be at high risk for substance misuse, and it can be difficult to cease taking drugs because stopping them enables old symptoms to recur but with more potency. There is little doubt that any drug, alcohol or tobacco can easily pass through the placenta into the developing foetus and cause harm.

Caffeine consumption

Over 70% of the UK population drink coffee, and the average consumption is two cups of coffee a day (International Communicaffe, 2021). The reasons for drinking coffee are often that it increases energy levels, alertness and overall wellbeing, and it is possible to tolerate high doses. These effects are useful if a parent needs to keep awake to tend to their infant. In low doses, caffeine is relatively safe; but larger doses can lead to problems with mental health.

Some parents prefer energy drinks as they contain high levels of caffeine which allows more to be consumed in smaller measures. This can result in caffeine intoxication. One study by Mikkelsen *et al.* (2017) found there were behavioural disorders in children at 11 years old if their mothers consumed high levels of coffee and tea when they were 15 weeks pregnant. It is thought that exposure to caffeine at this time may affect the unborn infant's brain.

Smoking

The dangers of smoking during pregnancy are well known and emphasised by practitioners working with pregnant women. Research has shown that smoking tobacco or marijuana, taking prescription pain relievers, or using illegal drugs during pregnancy is associated with double or even triple the risk of stillbirth (Wendell, 2013).

A rising number of adolescents are smoking cannabis, with a substantial upsurge in the amount of cannabis being consumed (Manthey *et al.*, 2021). Cannabis use is approximately 2.5 times more common amongst those who suffer from anxiety and depression (RCP & RCPsych, 2013). One study found that those who smoked cannabis have a higher risk of developing depression and suicidal behaviour in later life (Gobbi *et al.*, 2019). In light of Wendell's research (2013), it is advisable to stop consuming cannabis at least six months prior to conceiving (Murphy *et al.*, 2018). The relationship between smoking cannabis during pregnancy and other pregnancy and childhood outcomes is unclear, with the exception that it is linked to lower birth weight in infants (Gunn *et al.*, 2016).

Alcohol misuse

Alcohol may be used as a way of self-medicating, particularly after a stressful day, and for some people the urge to drink alcohol can be overwhelming. Alcohol misuse has a bi-directional relationship with depression, and parents may have co-existing issues with alcohol dependence and depression. The one issue increases the risk of the other, and as a result they can each make the other worse. Unfortunately, drinking can interfere with the recovery process from depression, as the more that is drunk, the worse the outcome, which means even moderate drinking can hinder any improvement in mood.

Excessive drinking can lead to a deficiency in the vitamin thiamine, which is important for brain function, including memory and reasoning. There are consequences for the baby in the womb, because high levels of consumption, particularly binge drinking, can result in a reduction in the infant's birth weight and, in a minority of cases, can be associated with foetal alcohol syndrome. This can cause lifetime problems for infants, including irreversible damage to their brain and bodily functions. Joint damage may affect mobility, and the infant may have difficulties with hearing and vision. The heart and kidneys may also be affected. However, an early diagnosis and support can make a positive difference.

There is evidence that even low-to-moderate drinking during pregnancy can have harmful effects on the foetus (Easey *et al.*, 2019). To add to this concern, it is now known that the children of mothers who drink alcohol during pregnancy may have an increased risk of developing depression themselves during adolescence (Easey, Timpson & Munafò, 2020).

Gambling addiction

Unlike some of the other pre-existing conditions parents may experience in the perinatal period, there may not be obvious signs of gambling addiction and it is therefore known as the 'hidden addiction' (Yorath, personal communication, 2021). Problem gambling not only impacts the affected parent but also the whole family, who may be reticent to talk about their relative's addiction due to shame and a perceived sense of stigma. As a result, relatively little is known about the harm gambling can cause.

Symptoms include the need to gamble to feel excitement; stopping gambling may cause a parent to feel restless and irritable. Loss of finances may motivate a parent to return to gambling habits, but they may lie to conceal their activities. They may depend on others to continue to spend money, and this can have an impact on relationships and the workplace. Parents with a gambling addiction may present with anxiety or depression, or physical symptoms such as migraines and stomach pains. They may also have other conditions including substance and alcohol misuse, unmanaged ADHD or bipolar disorder, and the original disorder will require treatment as well as their gambling problem.

If a parent has a known gambling addiction during the perinatal period, it is important for practitioners to recognise this and support the management of the parent's anxiety.

Interventions for maladaptive coping mechanisms

There are several ways that practitioners can support parents to ascertain what is happening in their life. They can identify parents' current coping strategies and offer approaches that may enable them to reduce their dependency on substances and alter their behavioural traits.

Parents who have been recognised as self-medicating or who have an addiction should ideally be referred to a specialist organisation where a treatment plan can be developed to identify the cause of the misuse, create achievable goals and define the objective to reach those goals. It is also important to tailor therapeutic interventions necessary to the type of misuse or addiction.

SUMMARY

It is important to explore the risk factors that a parent might have experienced, or is currently undergoing, to understand how and why circumstances may be affecting their mental health. It is equally important to determine any positive protective factors, and to support the parent to consider the options they have to maintain or improve their mental health. This can be essential if the parent is having difficulty in breastfeeding or is unaware of the value of skin-to-skin contact.

USEFUL RESOURCES

Perinatal mental health websites

Adfam provides support for practitioners and parents who are affected by substance misuse: https://adfam.org.uk

Best Beginnings has excellent resources on childcare for both parents and practitioners: www.bestbeginnings.org.uk

Birth Trauma Association supports practitioners and parents affected by birth trauma or loss: https://birthtraumaassociation.org

Dad Pad is a resource with information for new fathers: https://thedadpad.co.uk/neonatal

Ginger Bread is a charity working with single parents: www.gingerbread.org.uk

Hub of Hope is a resource enabling you to search for local services for support with most mental health conditions: https://hubofhope.co.uk

Maternal Mental Health Alliance is a charity with 120 organisations, dedicated to ensuring all women and families impacted by perinatal mental health problems have access to high-quality, compassionate care and support: https://maternalmentalhealthalliance.org

MIND is a mental health charity dedicated to helping parents with mental health conditions: www.mind.org.uk/information-support/guides-to-support-and-services/crisis-services/helplines-listening-services

NHS Mental Health Helplines are dedicated to supporting people experiencing mental health conditions: www.nhs.uk/mental-health/nhs-voluntary-charity-services/nhs-services

NHS talking therapies for anxiety and depression: www.nhs.uk/mental-health/talking-therapies-medicine-treatments/talking-therapies-and-counselling/nhs-talking-therapies

Domestic Violence websites

https://refuge.org.uk

http://respect.uk.net

NHS Perinatal mental health team

England: www.england.nhs.uk/mental-health/perinatal

Scotland: www.pmhn.scot.nhs.uk

Wales: https://bcuhb.nhs.wales/services/hospital-services/mental-health/perinatal-mental-health

Podcasts

The Royal College of Psychiatrists has produced a series of podcasts on mental health conditions. These can be found at: www.rcpsych.ac.uk/news-and-features/podcasts

CHAPTER-SPECIFIC WORKSHEETS FOR PRACTITIONERS (SEE APPENDIX)

Worksheet 5: Lifestyle choices in the perinatal period

Worksheet 6: Interactions between mood and lifestyle

Worksheet 9: Partner support

BREAKOUT: Considering neurodiversity in the perinatal period

Neurodivergence is a non-medical term which describes differences in the ways people's brains function. Neurodivergent people may think, communicate and behave in different ways to neurotypical people but, just like neurotypical people, they are all individuals who experience their own distinct strengths and challenges.

The main recognised neurodivergent conditions are:

- attention deficit hyperactivity disorder (ADHD)
- autism spectrum disorder (ASD)
- dyslexia
- dyspraxia.

It is important for practitioners to consider neurodivergent conditions during the perinatal period because some neurodivergent parents may experience extra challenges at this time. Practitioners should also be aware of how to adapt their practice to meet the needs of the neurodivergent person. This is becoming more relevant, as more adults are being diagnosed as neurodivergent.

Self-blame and anxiety, coupled with other depressive feelings, can demotivate neurodivergent parents from interacting with friends, family, health and support systems. As a result, they may withdraw socially. This has implications for supportive care for both the parent and the infant as the parent may feel they are not able to access the help they need. Having a clear understanding of neurodivergent conditions can help practitioners to tailor support and care to the individual's needs to ensure the best possible outcomes for both the parent and the infant. Like all parents, some parents with a neurodivergent condition will manage well during the perinatal period, while others may find it more challenging and need supportive interventions.

Making simple changes to the environment, or how communication takes place, can help to support neurodivergent parents. It is important to be mindful of the impact loud or different sounds and lighting may have on an autistic parent's comfort and, therefore, ability to concentrate.

Being patient and taking the time to listen to the parent can also help them to know that the practitioner understands the challenges they may experience when trying to explain how their infant is behaving or when they are indicating the type of help they would like to receive. Some parents may benefit from extra therapeutic interventions and, in some cases, medication.

The recommendations in Figure 3.1 were put together from a systematic review of the literature for supportive care for neurodivergent parents (Elliott, Buchanan & Bayes, 2024).

ADHD: For further information on ADHD, the ADHD Foundation is an integrated health and education service providing information and further signposting: www.adhdfoundation.org.uk

Autism: The National Autistic Society is doing great work helping to transform parents' lives and change attitudes to create a society that works for autistic people: www.autism.org.uk

JOURNEY MAP: RECOMMENDATIONS FROM THE SYSTEMATIC REVIEW OF LITERATURE

Navigating the Neurodivergent Perinatal Journey

ANTENATAL – PREPARING THE PATH

ASSESS NEEDS: Provide frequent check-ins; inquire about mood; co-create personalised plans and support informed choice; allow time for processing, use pauses and offer written summaries or recordings of visits.

SENSORY SUPPORT: Create calm environments; adjust lighting and noise levels.

SUPPORT EXECUTIVE FUNCTIONING: Use reminders, clear instructions, visual aids and role-play scenarios.

Key Focus: Understanding and Communication

LABOUR & BIRTH – NAVIGATE THE EXPERIENCE

SUPPORT PAIN MANAGEMENT: Acknowledge reported pain; encourage a birth plan considering sensory needs.

CONTINUITY: Familiar caregivers; sensory-friendly environments and minimise over-stimulation; support sensory preferences like movement, massage, water, scents, personal items, ear defenders and music.

ADDITIONAL SUPPORT: Incorporate vagus nerve techniques; provide anxiety support and maintain a non-judgemental atmosphere.

Key Focus: Comfort and Empowerment

POSTNATAL – EMBRACING THE TRANSITION

LACTATION: Ask permission before touch; support sensitivities; use clear, literal instructions; show videos and prepare antenatally.

CONTINUITY: Use familiar caregivers; consider home visits, doula support and create a plan.

EDUCATION: Offer information in various formats – role-play verbal, written demonstrations, videos and podcasts.

BONDING: Encourage skin-to-skin contact (not limited to the chest).

Key Focus: Adaptation and Support

CONTINUITY OF CARE – SUSTAINING THE CONNECTION

EXECUTIVE FUNCTION SUPPORT: Use organisational tools, visual schedules and written contacts/support lines; plan next steps clearly.

INFORMAL SUPPORT: Engage family/community; create a support-seeking plan and connect with resources.

CONTINUITY: Limit new caregiver introductions.

Key Focus: Long-term Support and Relationship Building

EMPOWERMENT AND ADVOCACY – OWNING THE JOURNEY

AUTONOMY: Support personalised birth plans; respect preferences, appreciate differences and encourage questions.

SELF-ADVOCACY: Offer resources for navigating health care.

EMPOWERMENT: Boost self-esteem; address fears with compassionate trauma-informed care; recognise strengths.

Key Focus: Advocacy and Personalisation

FINAL NOTE

INTERSECTIONALITY

Culturally Sensitive Care: Respect differences in gender, race and socio-economic status; address systemic barriers and advocate for resources like language access and financial support.

Source: Jata K. Elliott, Kate Buchanan, Sara Bayes, The neurodivergent perinatal experience—A systematic literature review on autism and attention deficit hyperactivity disorder. Image reproduced under a Creative Commons License 4.0 https://creativecommons.org/licenses/by/4.0/

FIGURE 3.1

Dyslexia: The British Dyslexia Association (BDA) can provide tools to make life easier for parents with dyslexia: www.bdadyslexia.org.uk

Dyspraxia: The Dyspraxia Foundation is a country-wide charity providing resources and support: https://dyspraxiauk.com/dyspraxia-foundation

RELEVANT WORKSHEETS FOR PRACTITIONERS

Worksheet 1: Pregnancy

Worksheet 3: The perinatal period

Worksheet 5: Lifestyle choices in the perinatal period

Worksheet 6: Interactions between mood and lifestyle

Worksheet 9: Partner support

CHAPTER 4

Mental Health Conditions Arising in the Perinatal Period

The antenatal period is significant for parents and the developing foetus, and any trauma experienced at this time can be destructive and detrimental to mental health. Several factors can affect the mental health of parents during this period; these include:

- becoming a parent as an adolescent (Siegel & Brandon, 2014)
- failure of contraceptives
- unplanned pregnancy, either accidental or planned by only one partner
- damaging relationships where parents are subjected to domestic violence
- ectopic pregnancy
- issues with infertility or pregnancy following in vitro fertilisation (IVF) (Lee *et al.*, 2011; Ross *et al.*, 2011)
- the physical and psychological impact of multiple pregnancies
- miscarriage or an abortion
- continuing with a pregnancy when a foetus may be affected by a genetic abnormality or a serious health condition.

Until fairly recently, parents have been reluctant to admit they had a mental health condition such as anxiety, depression or post-traumatic stress disorder (PTSD). However, it is now perfectly normal to talk about feelings, whether they be happy or sad. These conditions occur relatively often during the perinatal period and can cause parents to experience low self-esteem, feel that they are a failure or believe that they will be unable to cope with the demands of caring for a baby. A fear of their infant being taken into care by health and social care professionals may deter some parents from expressing their feelings and experiences to practitioners, so practitioners must apply their skills and expertise to determine whether the parent is unwell and, if so, how much intervention and support they require.

This chapter outlines the symptoms of some of the mental health conditions that parents may experience in the perinatal period, and it also suggests approaches that practitioners may take to support parents with these conditions.

PERINATAL ANXIETY

Anxiety is often characterised as the parent's excessive worry or fear about their perceived stressful events in their life. The 'fight-or-flight' action, caused by stress, is an important physical response that can keep the body safe from external harmful stimuli. This is particularly important for the pregnant mother as she needs to be able to keep her baby safe and protect it from harm by reacting quickly to avoid dangerous circumstances or to confront threatening situations (Goldfarb, 2019). In the short term, this stress can enhance memory, promoting the immediate recall of information around the time of the stressful encounter, and improve alertness. However, chronic stress has a more detrimental effect on the body: it can cause both acute and long-term changes in certain areas in the brain, which can lead to long-term physical and psychological damage, which in turn can affect the developing foetus.

Some parents with perinatal anxiety may have had pre-existing anxiety; this is often exacerbated by the added responsibility of pregnancy or caring for an infant.

Symptoms of anxiety

Some classic signs of anxiety are relatively straightforward to identify and diagnose; these include sweaty palms, agitation and difficulty concentrating. However, as symptoms can be physical, emotional and behavioural, sometimes it is difficult to determine whether a mother or father is suffering from anxiety without careful scrutiny. Physical symptoms of anxiety include:

- cardiovascular problems such as palpitations or feeling as if the heart is beating rapidly – can culminate in chest pains that often feel quite severe and can occur without warning

- compromised respiratory system because a parent is hyperventilating (breathing quickly and not absorbing sufficient oxygen) – can lead to shortness of breath and the sensation of panic

- neurological issues, partly associated with the cardiovascular and respiratory problems outlined – may include dizziness, dull and sometimes persistent headaches (which are not resolved by painkillers) and tingling or numbness in the fingers.

- sweating on the forehead or palm

- gastrointestinal symptoms (e.g. a dry mouth, nausea, an unsettled tummy) – can affect appetite, so parents may be reluctant to eat properly, preferring to snack on foods that are high in sugar and fat

- frequent micturition and bowel movements and (less

commonly) vomiting in pregnancy – can be related to perinatal anxiety

- disrupted sleep patterns and difficulties falling asleep, even though parents may be exhausted

- lethargy and a sense of dread – parents may feel that every bone in their body aches or that the wider world feels frightening.

Emotional and behavioural symptoms of anxiety include:

- feeling on edge or nervous all the time
- worrying excessively, even without rational cause
- difficulty concentrating and making decisions
- struggling to remember things
- feeling irritable and angry.

For parents who haven't previously struggled to cope with the demands of their day-to-day lives or were once meticulously organised, experiencing these challenging symptoms can lead to feelings of distress, inadequacy, irritability and anger.

Identifying perinatal anxiety

It is important to note that, as with all symptoms, physical causes must be ruled out before determining that a parent is exhibiting signs of anxiety.

Avoiding antenatal and well-baby clinics can be a sign of perinatal anxiety as parents may feel that they are being judged by health professionals; this feeling is compounded by sharing a waiting room with other parents who appear to be enjoying parenthood and look capable. A cycle of avoidance and social isolation can begin as their lack of contact widens the gap in their self-esteem (Fried *et al.*, 2020).

When someone is very stressed and exhibits some or most of the signs mentioned, the last thing they may want to do is to socialise and be forced to pretend they are in control of parenthood and their work–life balance. It is easier for them to avoid social situations and decline invitations with gatherings of friends and family. This isolation can lead to further loneliness, and the more a parent refuses to join in, the harder it can become for them to remain in contact with their social scene. Therefore, isolation and withdrawal from activities may be a way to identify anxiety in a parent.

There is a significant difference between typical feelings of stress and worry, experienced by many people at low levels, and suffering from anxiety. The clue is in the word 'suffering': anxious parents really are suffering due to their symptoms. A mother or father may have been diagnosed with anxiety following the conception of their infant and learned to cope with their feelings antenatally, but the added responsibility of caring for an infant in the postnatal period has the potential to exacerbate their symptoms.

Support strategies for parents with pre-existing anxiety in the perinatal period

Acknowledging that a parent is suffering from an anxiety state is the first step to supporting them. Listening and responding to their concerns can have great benefits. Someone who was already living with anxiety before becoming a parent may be knowledgeable about support and relaxation strategies that work for them – listen to the parent's experience and signpost them to how this support can be accessed.

Early recognition of the signs and symptoms of pre-existing anxiety resurfacing can prevent more serious problems developing. When a parent is allowed space and time to talk about how they are feeling, this enables both their mind and body to manage their anxiety more effectively. A parent can be helped to identify their emotional reactions, why they occur and why stress is caused. With milder anxiety, with support and by learning relaxation techniques a parent can learn to lessen these feelings. Many approaches can be used to promote relaxation, but practice and having the support to sustain calming practices is important. When the mind is at peace, it is more active and able to think logically. This allows a parent to have greater focus and to solve their problems and make decisions more easily. In cases where a parent previously accessed and benefited from support such as counselling or medication, and felt anxiety to have been resolved, they may welcome referral to healthcare services again and information about specialised support for the perinatal period.

Tokophobia

Parents, particularly mothers, may suffer from tokophobia, which is an extreme fear of childbirth. The cause of this fear is unclear, but a mother with tokophobia can dread getting pregnant, and if she does, she may want to avoid labour and vaginal birth, preferring to have an elective caesarean (Hofberg & Brockington, 2000).

Support strategies for parents experiencing perinatal anxiety

The first step is for a parent to acknowledge that they feel anxious. Talking with a parent in a non-judgemental way can help them express how they really feel, and this process can reveal simple solutions to problems that might cause a parent to feel overwhelmed. Exploring lifestyle choices will help, such as ensuring a parent has a nutritious diet and is avoiding alcohol and recreational drugs. Practitioners can also encourage parents to take regular exercise: going on walks or joining a gym may help. Breathing exercises and mindfulness can also be beneficial. If there is a support group in the area, a parent can be referred to them, as talking with other parents can be constructive. Other options include medication, which is prescribed by a clinician, or talking therapies, which are some of the most effective treatments. Referral to a cognitive behavioural therapist in a specialist perinatal mental health team may be helpful for some parents as CBT can have long-lasting effects.

PERINATAL POST-TRAUMATIC STRESS DISORDER (PTSD)

The amygdala, deep inside the limbic system, is the part of the brain that activates the automatic stress response. This is the fight-or-flight response: the brain's automatic physiological reaction to something that is stressful or frightening. The amygdala is the oldest, most primitive part of the brain, and it cannot distinguish between a real threat and a perceived or imagined threat (Rajmohan & Mohandas, 2007). The limbic system is sometimes known as the emotional brain, and it has a major role in the experience and expression of emotions. PTSD has only recently been associated with the perinatal period and the trauma that mothers may have experienced during the labour and delivery of their infant. Trauma may be caused by different factors, from experiencing surgical interventions to the fear of losing the infant. Relatively recently, awareness has grown that fathers can also suffer from PTSD due to experiencing the same situation as the mother and feeling that they are unable to control it.

When memories of traumatic events are triggered, a parent may feel as if the event is happening again at that time. They feel as though the threat is present and the fear response system is triggered again, which means the amygdala is switched on to high response.

The lasting effects of reactions to traumatic, stressful experiences are called post-traumatic symptoms (Alder *et al.*, 2006). PTSD is often associated with symptoms of depression and anxiety (Auxéméry, 2018). PTSD symptoms can be categorised into three types:

- intrusive symptoms (associated with the mind)
  - intrusive memories of a traumatic event.
  - flashbacks – feeling as though an event is being re-experienced

- hyper-arousal/fear response (associated with the body):
  - difficulties with sleep.
  - difficulties with concentration

  - an exaggerated startle response in reaction to triggers related to previous trauma
  - physical symptoms of anxiety such as sweating and shaking

- avoidance behaviours
  - active or passive avoidance of triggering environments – a parent who has experienced trauma in a clinical setting may avoid hospital or clinic appointments.

PTSD related to childbirth

Although parents may have attended antenatal classes and feel they are fully aware of what happens during the delivery of their infant, some may still feel unprepared for their birth experience. It has been reported by the National Childbirth Trust that as many as one in three parents feel traumatised after giving birth (NCT, 2023). Sometimes labour is longer and more intense than parents anticipate, leading to unplanned surgical interventions or emergency surgery. Some fathers have witnessed their partner and child's lives being at risk during childbirth, feeling powerless to offer support as health professionals intervened (Etheridge & Slade, 2017).

Some fathers have experienced PTSD symptoms, such as repeated nightmares and negative mood swings, several months following the birth of their infant. Other fathers have reported that they have struggled with their emotions towards the infant, inadvertently blaming them for their partner's distress (Daniels *et al.*, 2020). Mothers who have symptoms of PTSD have experienced anxiety attacks and poor sleep patterns due to worrying that they would become pregnant again (Greenfield, Jomeen & Glover, 2019). These fears have been so invasive that some parents have taken steps to avoid having sex to prevent further pregnancies as a precaution against having to endure similar experiences of trauma (Byrne *et al.*, 2017). Some practitioners may underestimate the impact of traumatic situations, or not recognise that trauma has occurred, and so fail to provide sufficient debriefing, leaving parents to process their fear or terror without professional support.

Support strategies for parents with perinatal PTSD

Recognising that a parent may be suffering from PTSD is an important first step. Asking a parent about their birth experiences is the best approach to finding out if they are experiencing symptoms of PTSD. Allow parents to speak freely about how they felt about labour and birth and validate their feelings by supporting them to mourn the birth process if it did not turn out as they had hoped and expected. Encourage them to stay active, eat well and enjoy the things they used to. Let them know that there are organisations that can help to lessen their feeling of despair and that they can be referred to a perinatal mental health specialist team or a general practitioner who can offer effective therapies.

Some practitioners are trained in eye movement desensitisation and reprocessing therapy (EMDR), which can be used when the parent has suffered from post-traumatic stress disorder. This therapy highlights the function of the brain in information processing. It conceptualises memories of trauma that have been insufficiently processed. The parent will be asked to move their eyes from side to side simultaneously to desensitise a traumatic memory and reprocess it into something more acceptable to them. This therapy is only available in some parts of the country and must be practised by an authorised therapist.

POSTNATAL DEPRESSION

One in seven mothers suffer from postnatal depression, which can occur at any time during the perinatal period (Carlson *et al.*, 2022). Some studies have shown that depressive symptoms can also occur within the antenatal period (Biaggi *et al.*, 2016; Heron *et al.*, 2004). Some symptoms are more obvious than others, but these are the most common:

- fatigue and feeling tired all the time

- depressed mood, present for most of the time
- loss of joy
- lethargy
- lack of interest or motivation
- difficulties sleeping, but not due to the demands of the infant
- vague aches and pains
- changes in appetite
- lack of sex drive
- self-neglect
- avoiding social situations
- feelings of worthlessness or guilt
- indecision and lack of concentration
- thoughts of suicide.

If it is not recognised or treated, postnatal depression can impair parent–infant bonding and can be associated with negative parenting practices and difficulties with breastfeeding. It may contribute to relationship problems and issues with an infant's physical and psychological development. Sleep deprivation, low mood and low interest in the things that they used to care about can profoundly affect a parent's ability to care for their infant and to enjoy aspects of parenthood.

Case study: Donna's experiences of postnatal depression

Donna had always been a vibrant character, the life and soul of the party. Nothing seemed to faze her. Donna became pregnant during a weekend away; she had previously not known the father of the child and was not planning to have a baby. After much thought, Donna decided to continue with the pregnancy. She felt she would have to give up her profession but was determined to remain in work as long as possible. Donna did not make the father aware of her pregnancy. Although she had many work colleagues, her only contact with them was on an online platform due to working from home.

At Donna's first scan, the sonographer's worried look told her something was wrong. Donna had to face the news that her baby would need specialist care once it was born. Although clinicians were sympathetic and offered information services, Donna felt very alone and anxious. Donna worried about the future and wondered what the outlook for herself and her child would be. She contemplated suicide.

No one suspected that Donna was experiencing issues with her mental health.

Reflection points:

- How could practitioners have identified that Donna was at risk of perinatal illness?
- What support strategies could a practitioner implement?

Support strategies for parents experiencing postnatal depression

Warning signs of postnatal depression may be difficult to detect, particularly if the parent resists acknowledging or is in denial about their symptoms. However, asking how they really feel about being a parent, their current environment and taking care to be non-judgemental about what the parent is saying can be very cathartic. It can lead to the parent having a greater understanding about how they feel and why they feel like that and can help to avert crisis situations.

Some conversation starters:

- 'I know everyone is focused on the baby, but I want to hear more about you.'[1]

---

1 Suggestion from the Moms' Mental Health Matters Conversation Starter Postcard, hosted by the National Child and Maternal Health Education Program https://www.nichd.nih.gov/ncmhep/materials/moms-conversation-postcard-txtalt

- 'Did you know that postnatal depression affects more than one in every ten women within a year of giving birth?'
- 'I really want to know how you're feeling, and I will listen to you.'
- 'Is there someone in your family or circle of friends who you can talk to about your feelings?'

There have been considerable changes in health and social care services to ensure that parents' mental health in the perinatal period is monitored and supported. However, supporting parents' wellbeing should not only be the responsibility of the practitioner, it should also be supported by families and society.

The use of assessment tools and pathways can help practitioners to screen parents for depressive symptoms. The Edinburgh Postnatal Depression Scale (EPDS) and PHQ-9 (Patient Hospital Questionnaire) are the most commonly used tools. The EPDS has also been validated for use with fathers and in the antenatal period. As with all assessment tools, they should not be used without adequate training. Further details about assessment tools can be found in Chapter 5. Patience and active listening will help parents who are suffering from depressive symptoms.

Practitioners can ensure that they ask parents how they are feeling each time they visit a parent's home or the parent attends clinic. The use of assessment tools can help to determine how a parent is feeling and will help the practitioner to discuss responses in greater depth. It may also be constructive to explore the parent's diet, activities and any self-medication, and it can be suggested that alcohol, smoking and recreational drugs are avoided.

For clinical or specialist support, parents can be referred to a general practitioner for medication or to a perinatal mental health team who can further assess parents' needs. Talking therapies are often effective for parents experiencing postnatal depression. A combination of antidepressants and talking therapy is often the most successful treatment. The best time to start supporting parents is at the very beginning of their infant's life, and practitioners can encourage all family members to be vigilant about the health and wellbeing of parents-to-be and new parents (Netsi *et al.*, 2018). The birth of the infant is also the birth of the parent.

Case study: Leroy's experiences of paternal depression

Leroy was a father of four, whose youngest had been born six months ago. Since the birth, Leroy had been struggling to sleep and eating badly, and his relationship with his wife had deteriorated to the point where they agreed to separate. On the advice of a health visitor, Leroy sought help from his GP, who diagnosed him with paternal depression and referred him to a specialist perinatal mental health counsellor.

Over time, with support from the counsellor, Leroy was able to reflect on his anxieties about himself and his capability as a father, and how they had fuelled arguments with his partner. He also came to understand the way his mental health difficulties and lack of self-care were acting as a cycle, and that eating better and looking after his physical wellbeing would make him more able to cope emotionally and support his wife.

Reflection points:

- What information could indicate that Leroy was struggling with depression, even if he did not talk about his feelings?
- Based on your knowledge from this book, how might signs of depression differ in a father to a mother?

BIPOLAR DISORDER

Once known as manic-depression, bipolar disorder has been brought to wider attention by several television programmes featuring characters who have the condition. In the soap opera *Eastenders*, two of the characters, a mother and daughter clearly display the symptoms of bipolar disorder when they are in crisis, and sensitively educate the audience about the challenges, barriers and stigma they face, as well as the joy and love conveyed through their personalities. Although either parent can have bipolar disorder, it is more likely that practitioners will come across mothers who have the condition. The onset of bipolar disorder may be rapid or insidious; it is often detected when someone's behaviour is so erratic that it becomes a serious cause for concern. Some parents may have been previously diagnosed with bipolar disorder, but childbirth can be a trigger for the illness (Jones & Craddock, 2005). Women with a family history of bipolar disorder, particularly a first-degree relative who has bipolar disorder, are more likely to be affected (Jones & Craddock, 2005). A first-degree relative is a family member, such as a brother, sister, parent or child, who shares about 50 percent of their genes with the mother.

Until recently, little was known about this condition, which primarily affects the brain and causes severe shifts in mood function. Bipolar means having two 'poles' or extremities and the opposite extreme from mania is depression. Sometimes, mood swings in bipolar disorder are dramatic; at other times there may be a slow decline in mood, resulting in depression. This can be a traumatic time for the mother as she ebbs and flows between the two 'poles', not knowing how she will react or how feelings will be interpreted. There is usually little insight or control into her behaviour; if there was, the mother would certainly have more control over her behaviour.

Bipolar disorder can present challenges for the mother and her interaction with her infant during the first year of life and may even present developmental risks. As this may have consequences for the infant, it is important that a diagnosis is established. This usually occurs during a manic episode, when the family are concerned about the mother's conduct and refer her to the GP. The symptoms of bipolar disorder include:

- difficulties with concentration
- extreme mania, which entails high energy levels
- fast and disorganised speech that reflects confused thought processes
- issues with communication that can cause parents with bipolar disorder to become irate, irritable or aggressive when other people fail to interpret what they mean.

The psychopathology of bipolar disorder can make mothers more vulnerable to impaired bonding with their infant (Boekhorst *et al.*, 2021). In some cases, a mother might engage in compulsive sexual behaviour during manic periods.

A mother may falsely believe, in a delusional state, that she is capable of anything, however unrealistic. For example, she may believe she has won the lottery and lavishly spend money she does not possess. In extreme cases this can lead to family debt. The feelings of euphoria are exhilarating, and for some, that feeling cannot be replicated by everyday life events.

Support strategies for parents experiencing bipolar disorder in the perinatal period

It is important to exclude other reasons for symptoms of bipolar disorder; for example, an organic cause or the use of mood-enhancing drugs. Any supportive and clinical interventions should address both the needs of the parents and their interactions with their infant. It has been suggested that it is prudent to help mothers to be more sensitive to their infant's cues and provide them with the skills to work in harmony with their infant's responses (Anke *et al.*, 2020). Patience, listening and responding are key to supporting mothers and fathers. Many parents with bipolar disorder will be under the care of a psychiatrist and are prescribed medication. Several medications can help to stabilise mood, but they need careful monitoring that requires regular blood tests. The condition cannot be cured but it can be effectively managed.

PERSONALITY DISORDER

A 'personality' is a collective combination of the characteristics or qualities that form a person's distinct character. Often, the term 'personality disorder' is poorly understood. The causes of personality disorder are complex but are likely to be a combination of early experiences, brain development and genetics. Some parents with borderline personality disorder were found to have been abused as children, and almost one third of maltreated children go on to develop the disorder. A significant number of infants born to mothers with personality disorder are disorganised in their attachment at the age of 13 months (Bozzatello *et al.*, 2021).

Parents with borderline personality disorder are characterised by persistent, fixed personality traits that can cause instability and difficulties interacting socially. Parents with the disorder are at greater risk of a wide range of psychological outcomes (American Psychiatric Association, 1994) and may face challenges during the perinatal period. Studies have suggested that their needs are often not heard or understood, and judgements are made about their parenting skills, with services struggling to support their complex needs (Prasad *et al.*, 2022; Zacharia *et al.*, 2020)

Challenges parents with a personality disorder may experience in the perinatal period

A parent with a personality disorder may have thoughts on how they view themselves, the world and others that are very different to those of others. They may have difficulties interacting with other people and find relationships hard to maintain because of the inappropriateness and intensity of their behaviour. Sometimes the parent's actions can be impulsive, which can be damaging and confusing for them, and may have consequences for others: for example, example, spending and losing money they may have borrowed and are unable to repay. Their approach to caring for their infant can 'oscillate between extreme forms of hostile control and passive aloofness' (Stepp *et al.*, 2012). It can be difficult to understand the parent's disruptive, upsetting behaviour. This can cause concern for the practitioner, particularly if the parent does not believe there is a problem. The way in which some infants are treated by parents with personality disorders means that they could be considered as a high-risk group (Stepp *et al.*, 2021).

Parents with personality disorders are more likely to misuse substances, deliberately self-harm and be known to social services because of the safeguarding risks associated with their behaviours. They may be exhausted by their experiences in the perinatal period and need significant support. Sometimes, parents are unable to recognise their escalating anxiety, and it is therefore the responsibility of family and friends to draw attention to the distress this may be causing both the parent and the infant.

Support strategies for parents with personality disorders

Practitioners can help parents and family to understand the conditions and the support and help that may be required to help them through the perinatal period. Parents can be referred to applied psychological services, where treatments may include mentalisation-based therapy, dialectical behaviour therapy or cognitive behavioural therapy (see Chapter 5 for more on psychological therapies). Clinicians can prescribe antipsychotic and antidepressant medication. As knowledge about the disorder increases, so does the awareness of the need for more appropriate services. Previously, practitioners may have been unsure which services to refer parents to, but now there are specialist perinatal mental health services that are able to help and support parents who have complex needs.

PUERPERAL PSYCHOSIS

Puerperal psychosis is a severe and rare mental health condition that can be frightening for mothers and their families. It affects one in

500 mothers; women with a history of psychosis or bipolar disorder have almost a 50% chance of the condition recurring, and the risk of puerperal psychosis is heightened if a first-degree relative has bipolar disorder (Davies, 2017; Perry *et al.*, 2019).

It can be difficult to determine if a mother is experiencing psychosis as some of the things she says may sound quite plausible. Psychosis affects all the senses: smell, sight, taste, sound and touch. It can also include paranoia, delusions and hallucinations, all of which are frightening, and for the mother they are perfectly believable.

Indicators that things may not be quite right include the mother being more energetic than usual, with her energy levels abnormally elevated, appearing to be unusually excited and very talkative, bordering on manic. There may be a tendency to not want to rest or purposefully remain awake whilst being vigilant over the care of her infant, even though she may be extremely tired. The mother's behaviours may give cause for concern as the mother might act as if she is apprehensive or suspicious that something dreadful is about to happen.

To the practitioner, none of this makes any sense, but there is little that can dissuade the mother of her beliefs as she is convinced that everything she hears, sees, smells, feels and tastes is dangerous and a threat. Examples of sensory symptoms of puerperal psychosis:

- Smell – the mother believes there is a (non-existent) gas leak and that someone is trying to harm her or blow up her house.

- Sight – the mother is frightened of a bizarre shape in the kitchen that she believes is trying to control her mind or has come to harm both her and her infant.

- Taste – the mother may complain that her food tastes odd and that someone is trying to poison her.

- Sound – the mother may hear voices threatening to harm her or warn her that the practitioner is there to harm her and her baby. Conversely, she may also believe that she is the saviour of the world and that her infant is blessed and needs to be revered. She may believe that soundwaves from her phone are sending her messages or controlling her mind.

- Touch –the mother believes that her constantly itchy skin is the result of creatures crawling over her body.

This is an example of a real experience of puerperal psychosis from the author Laura Dockrill's book *What Have I Done: Motherhood, Mental Illness and Me* (2021):

> After Jet was born, I had quietly become convinced that [my partner's] dad was judging me. That he didn't like me. The negative delusions and paranoia about him came on thick and fast and took a very long time to lift.
>
> I decided, in my delusion, that on that night before I was admitted to the psychiatric hospital, he had deliberately played this intense classical music to put me under a spell. I believed – in my psychosis – that he was performing some kind of self-taught shock-treatment hypnosis therapy, a sort of home-baked lie detector/interrogation/torture process. In my mind, he had taken off his glasses and stared me straight in the eye. His eyes were like a microscope lens. He was dissecting me.

Support strategies for mothers experiencing puerperal psychosis

The mother requires attention, and medical help should be summoned immediately. The hallucinations and delusions may last for many weeks, but the appropriate medication will eradicate them in time. It is also possible that the cause is organic and results from infection, drug use, or abnormal levels of blood glucose, which may alter the brain chemistry and lower the levels of dopamine.

Case study: Theresa and Tom's experiences of puerperal psychosis and paternal depression

Theresa and Tom were excited about the birth of their second child and had everything planned. Theresa had been previously diagnosed with bipolar disorder, and during her teens, she had been so poorly that she had been sectioned under the Mental Health Act. Since then, Theresa had managed her illness with medication and by attending an online self-help group. Tom was fully aware of Theresa's condition and knew how and when her mental health was deteriorating.

Unfortunately, the birth of their second daughter was traumatic and overwhelming for both parents. Theresa remained in hospital for a few days before being discharged. While the midwife was making a home visit she noticed that Theresa was acting strangely. Theresa was reluctant to carry her daughter out of her cot to be examined, saying the girl was sent by Jesus and must be untouched. Theresa then looked into the distance and started laughing. When the midwife asked Theresa what she was laughing about, she said the angels were singing to her, and she could see them waving their wings above her head, showering her with stardust. The midwife instantly realised that Theresa was ill. She immediately referred her to the GP and perinatal mental health specialist services. Theresa was admitted to a mother and baby unit 70 miles away from her home.

This had a significant impact on Tom who was struggling with his own mental health as well as caring for his elder daughter. He had no one to speak to about his experience of seeing his wife endure a traumatic birth. He was also aware that he did not have the time to bond with his new daughter. For the first time in his life, Tom felt alone, he had no family to help, and Theresa's family lived in Spain. He had always been independent and did not feel it was right to ask for any help, so he tried to cope on his own. However, the stress of looking after his daughter and his ruminating thoughts lowered his mood. Tom had to cease his normal activities; he stopped going to the gym and meeting friends. For the first time in his life, Tom felt suicidal.

Tom told no one about his challenging experiences of loneliness and not knowing what to do for the best for his wife and infant until his third child was due to be born. During this time a specialist perinatal mental health service had been commissioned, and as new parents, both Tom and Theresa were offered an assessment of their mental health. Although Tom felt he could not be honest, the practitioner inquired about his previous experiences and Tom felt he had no alternative but to express how he had been expected to cope alone and how he had been badly let down by perinatal services. The practitioner was surprised but sympathetic. She listened to Tom as he poured out how he felt alone when every service seemed to focus on Theresa, and no one even bothered to ask how he was doing. He explained that he felt that the system treated him as a spare part rather than as a part of his family. He did not resent the attention on Theresa and wanted her to receive the treatment she deserved. Tom felt he could have been so much better as a father if only he had been given the chance. He had 'let down' his family, and he wanted to ensure things were different this time.

The practitioner recognised Tom's situation and told him that the services had become more aware of the impact the perinatal period had on fathers' mental health and, as a result, were now more involved with their care too. The practitioner offered Tom an assessment tool which allowed him the opportunity to write down how he felt. The practitioner took the time to explore all the questions and the responses Tom gave. The practitioner asked why his wife had been ill and what her treatment entailed. The practitioner encouraged Tom to write down any questions he had, and he was also referred to a fathers' group and online resources.

Reflection points:

- What signs could indicate that a parent may be experiencing psychosis?
- How could a practitioner respond to a parent reporting delusions?
- What advice would you signpost to the partner of the parent?

Support strategies for families in which the mother has puerperal psychosis

Mothers with puerperal psychosis should be referred to a general practitioner as a medical emergency. After recovery, both parents should be supported by the perinatal mental health team to ensure they are coping, and their needs are addressed. The team could refer the parent to the specialist psychologist or social worker. The parent could also be directed to a support group or advised of a suitable online service.

OBSESSIVE COMPULSIVE DISORDER (OCD)

Estimates vary, but about 1–3% of all people will experience OCD during their lifetime (Brock, Rizvy & Hany, 2025). Around 1 in 50 mothers have OCD during pregnancy (Tommy's n.d.).

OCD has often been associated with people who are obsessive about cleanliness around the home, fearful of germs and contamination, and who tidy up frequently, but this is not a full picture of OCD. As previously stated, OCD is characterised by three main parts:

- 'Obsessions – frequent unpleasant thoughts, images, urges or doubts
- Anxiety – distress caused by these unpleasant thoughts
- Compulsions – behaviours like washing hands or mental acts such as counting, that the person keeps repeating, to try to reduce their anxiety or to prevent bad things from happening.' (Wales Mental Health Network, 2023)

However, it is often a hidden disorder, with intrusive thoughts causing distress. Some OCD-related behaviours cannot always be readily observed.

Parents may feel high levels of anxiety in talking about their feelings with a health professional and may be worried about the consequences of disclosing that they are experiencing obsessive thoughts. They may fear judgement, particularly if their thoughts involve worry about causing harm to their child. If a parent discusses OCD symptoms, let them know this is a common mental health problem and be reassuring. Let them know that there is effective treatment available.

Challenges that parents with OCD may experience in the perinatal period

The perinatal period is a vulnerable time, with increased responsibilities for the parent now that they are looking after a baby.

Everybody experiences intrusive thoughts, but in OCD thoughts create distress and become obsessive. These can then lead to compulsions that negatively affect quality of life. In perinatal OCD, it is common for obsessions and compulsions to centre on the baby, often on cleanliness or fears of contamination. For example, failure to ensure an infant is scrupulously clean could falsely be viewed by the parent as neglect, or they worry that their child will become ill through contact with germs.

A parent with OCD may be excessively motivated to try and keep their infant safe at all times. Of course, all parents want to protect their children, but in OCD the perceived threat is greater than the reality. They may also experience obsessive thoughts that they may cause harm to their child. People with OCD don't become violent or act on these thoughts, but the worry feels real to the parent (Shah, 2025).

The parent may be unable to stop compulsive behaviours, sometimes to the detriment of their own health. For example, they may excessively wash milk bottles and the infant's clothes, ensuring the infant's outfits are frequently changed for fear of contamination from spilt liquids or foods. They feel severe anxiety, and it is possible that the parent will exhibit the signs and symptoms of similar anxiety disorders, such as feeling anxious all the time, worrying about the slightest thing, avoiding social situations, problems with sleeping or eating, and feeling on edge. A parent with OCD may believe that completing the tasks will alleviate their symptoms, whereas in reality it exacerbates them as compulsive actions lead to a cycle (Figure 4.1).

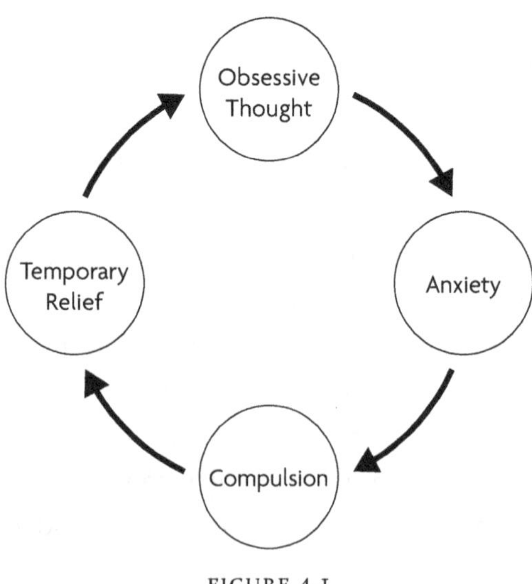

FIGURE 4.1

If these behaviours are ignored or left untreated, it can seriously interfere with daily living, as these compulsions take precedence. In some cases where the parent has extreme fears of harming their child, they may begin to avoid them, which of course affects their attachment and relationship.

Support strategies for parents with pre-existing OCD during the perinatal period

The parents may be aware they have OCD and have used previous coping strategies to help with their wellbeing. The practitioner could help the parent to recollect what approaches they used to relax and to feel less anxious. Listening to the parents' concerns and helping to support them by understanding their behaviours can reduce the parents' fears and help them to understand how some of their activities can be irrational.

Support for perinatal OCD

Listening to the parents' concerns and helping to support them by signposting them to support so they can get appropriate treatment is vital. Treatment is generally:

- CBT
- CBT with exposure and response prevention
- medication.

SUMMARY

There is an increasing awareness of perinatal mental health disorders, yet some parents have suggested that their symptoms have been missed or marginalised by some health professionals. A sound knowledge of any previous mental health issues would help the practitioner to understand why the parent is feeling as they do. Ensuring there are robust assessment strategies in place to identify any signs of a mental health disorder is important to help the practitioner explore the impact of them with the parent. This will help the parent have a greater understanding of their thoughts and emotions and how this makes them feel towards themselves and their infant.

Once recognised and assessed, parents experiencing mental health conditions can be supported in ways that enable them to function and cope. Practitioners can help parents to reduce their anxiety, and there are many effective parenting support programmes. Simple stress relievers can also help parents to understand their feelings and teach them how to manage their own wellbeing, which will positively affect their infant.

USEFUL RESOURCES

Bipolar disorder

For further information contact Bipolar UK, the only national charity dedicated to empowering individuals and families affected by bipolar disorder. Peer support is at the core of their work: www.bipolaruk.org

General perinatal mental health support

The Hub of Hope is the UK's leading mental health support database. It is provided by national mental health charity, Chasing the Stigma, and brings local, national, peer, community, charity, private and NHS mental health support and services together in one place for the first time: https://hubofhope.co.uk

The Maternal Mental Health Alliance (MMHA) is a UK-wide charity and network of over 100 organisations dedicated to ensuring that women and families affected by perinatal mental health problems have access to high-quality, comprehensive perinatal mental health care and support: https://maternalmentalhealthalliance.org

PTSD

For further information, PTSD UK is the only UK-based charity dedicated to raising awareness of post-traumatic stress disorder: www.ptsduk.org

Puerperal psychosis

Action on Postpartum Psychosis: www.app-network.org

OCD

Maternal OCD: https://maternalocd.org

CHAPTER-SPECIFIC WORKSHEETS FOR PRACTITIONERS (SEE APPENDIX)

Worksheet 1: Pregnancy

Worksheet 3: The perinatal period

Worksheet 5: Lifestyle choices in the perinatal period

Worksheet 6: Interactions between mood and lifestyle

Worksheet 8: Thoughts, feelings and behaviours

CHAPTER 5

Assessment and Therapeutic Interventions

ASSESSMENT

Screening parents for depression and anxiety during the perinatal period, as well as finding out if they have a history of experiencing a mental health condition, can enable practitioners to tailor parents' treatment to their needs and help them to bond with their infant. Assessment tools include the PHQ-9 (Sidebottom *et al.*, 2012) and CORE 10 (Barkham *et al.*, 2012). Details of these assessments, together with the forms can be found online. The assessment questions in these screening tools are similar to the Edinburgh Postnatal Depression Scale (EPDS: Cox & Holden, 2003). The EPDS assessment tool can be located online; it is free to use provided all photocopies cite full accreditation to the authors.

The prerequisite for developing a high standard of practice in assessing parents' needs is to ensure that forms are completed in a culturally sensitive manner, with an awareness of a parent's level of education and literacy, and an acknowledgement of any visual or hearing impairments. For some parents, reading English may be difficult and it may be necessary to work with a translator (Cox, Holden & Henshaw, 2014).

Few parents report finding assessment questions intrusive, and the majority welcome the opportunity to discuss how they are really feeling. Parents have the opportunity to write down and discuss how they feel, and it is important that practitioners go through questionnaires with parents to ensure that each question is understood and agreed. However, it is also important to be aware that some parents may fear that if they reveal their true feelings, this will be viewed as a cause for concern and a practitioner will consider taking their infant into care. Practitioners must therefore be sensitive to the reticence of some parents to share their emotions and take the time to non-judgementally find out about their experiences before signposting them to appropriate support.

The EPDS

The EPDS was introduced nearly 40 years ago. It was devised by psychiatrist Professor John Cox, health visitor and psychologist Jenny Holden and psychiatrist Dr Ruth Sagovsky (Cox *et al.*, 1987). It has been cited over 12,000 times and is highly regarded by many researchers, clinicians and practitioners who believe that – through careful interpretation – it can provide a sound indication of how a parent may be feeling.

This tool was originally designed to recognise depression, as postnatal depression was the most frequently diagnosed postnatal mental illness. However, it is now recognised that some of the questions relate to anxiety, so responses can also indicate if a parent is feeling anxious. As with the introduction of any assessment tool, the practitioner needs training in the use of the EPDS to administer it correctly. A paper copy is given to the parent in the presence of the practitioner and handed back to be 'scored'. The scoring process is not onerous and is designed to give practitioners a clear indication of how a parent is feeling and has been feeling over the past two weeks.

There are ten screening questions that can show whether a parent has symptoms common in those who have anxiety and depression during pregnancy and up to 12 months following childbirth. Ideally, the EPDS should be completed in a calm environment. The parent should be allowed the freedom to talk without anyone else present.

It is not intended to provide a diagnosis, and it relies on the competence of the practitioner to decide, with the parent, the most appropriate resources, signposting and resources.

Each of the ten questions on the form requires an answer that comes closest to reflecting how the parent has felt during the past seven days. Each answer has a score, and the total score is calculated by adding the numbers selected for each of the ten questions. If the score is above 12, the practitioner will go through the individual questions to determine why the parent responded the way they did. It is, however, in all cases, important to go through the whole form with the parent to ensure they understand the questions and have responded appropriately.

The EPDS questions

Several of the questions relate to depression, and high-scoring answers may indicate a depressive state. For example:

Question 1 presents the statement 'I have been able to laugh and see the funny side of things.' The possible answers are:

1. As much as I always could (which scores 0).
2. Not quite so much now (which scores 1).
3. Definitely not so much now (which scores 2).
4. No, not at all (which scores 3).

Question 2 presents the statement: 'I have looked forward with enjoyment to things.' The possible answers are:

1. As much as I ever did (which scores 0).
2. Rather less than I used to (which scores 1).
3. Definitely less than I used to (which scores 2).
4. Hardly at all (which scores 3).

However, some of the EPDS questions may be more relevant to anxiety. For example:

Question 3 presents the statement: 'I have blamed myself unnecessarily when things have gone wrong.' The possible answers are:

1. Yes some of the time (which scores 3)
2. Yes most of the time (which scores 2).
3. Not very often (which scores 1).
4. No, not ever (which scores 0).

Question 4 presents the statement: 'I have been anxious or worried for no good reason.' The possible answers are:

1. No not at all (which scores 0).
2. Hardly ever (which scores 1).
3. Yes sometimes (which scores 2).
4. Yes very often (which scores 3).

Examining the possible answers, the less depressed the parent appears, the lower the score. When considering the signs and symptoms of depression, the depressed parent is more likely to say, 'Definitely less than I used to' or 'Hardly at all'. The answers reflect what the parent is feeling, and it is the responsibility of the practitioner to explore the reasons for the parent's responses and to follow up by asking the parent if they can think of reasons why they 'hardly look forward to anything'. The parent may admit they are exhausted, reticent about socialising and with little energy to participate in events. All of which, as discussed, can be indicators of depressive symptoms.

Question 7 presents the statement: 'I have been so unhappy I have difficulty in sleeping.' The possible answers are:

1. Yes, most of the time (which scores 3).

2. Yes, sometimes (which scores 2).
3. No, not very often (which scores 1).
4. No, not at all (which scores 0).

Having difficulty sleeping is common, however, in the context of this question sleep difficulties are not those caused by an unsettled infant or by social commitments. The key words are 'so unhappy', indicating that the parent's mood has interfered with their sleep. This affords the practitioner an opportunity to elicit what is causing the parent's unhappiness and why it is affecting their sleep.

Question 10 presents the statement: 'The thought of harming myself has occurred to me.' The possible answers are:

1. Yes quite often (which scores 3).
2. Sometimes (which scores 2).
3. Hardly ever (which scores 1).
4. Never (which scores 0).

This is a sensitive question, and it can sometimes be easy to dismiss the parent's answers by suggesting that the parent 'does not really mean that' or that they are 'being silly'. However, responses should always be taken seriously and given careful consideration. The parent may misinterpret the question and may not assume it refers to thoughts of suicide. For some, their thoughts may be fleeting, lasting only a few hours, or on a repetitive cycle, but for others, time is spent contemplating the way in which they would harm themselves permanently. Having an infant is not always a protective factor, and a seriously depressed parent may perceive that harming themselves will protect their family from their illness and related behaviour. It is important never to underestimate the risk of suicide in the perinatal period.

Assessing fathers' needs

A model of care has been developed called the Hanwill Model (MMHA, 2020; see Figure 5.1), which outlines a pathway of care that can be used for parents to ensure they have the correct access to the support they need. Along with using the EPDS, or other assessment tools, it may be pertinent to ask questions about the father's behaviours, which may be affecting the way he feels. For example:

- Do you feel that you are consuming more alcohol since the pregnancy or after the birth of your child?
- Do you think you are avoiding situations more than usual?
- How does this make you feel?

Answers can lead to a fuller conversation about the reasons motivating potential damaging behaviours and provide practitioners with a fuller sense of the father's experiences.

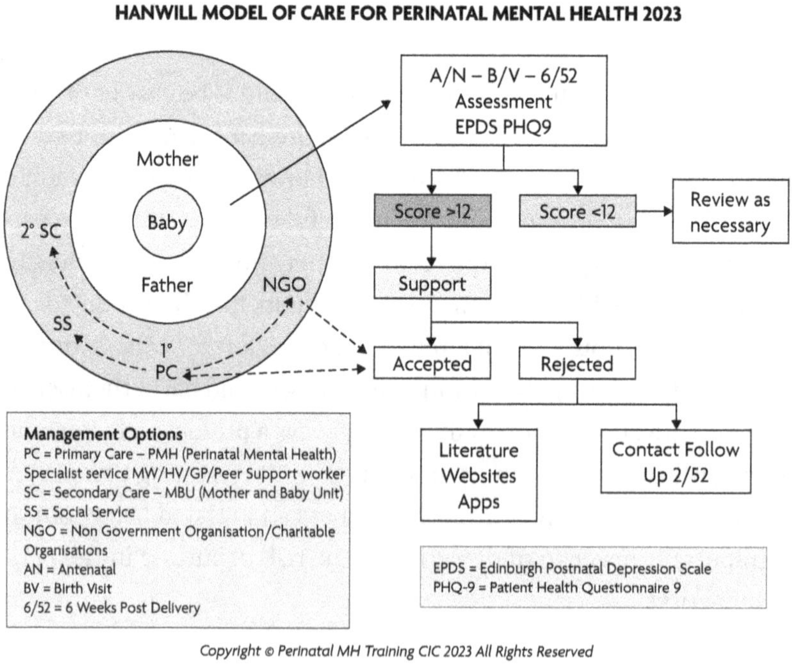
HANWILL MODEL OF CARE FOR PERINATAL MENTAL HEALTH 2023
Mother
Baby
Father
2° SC
SS
1° PC
NGO
A/N – B/V – 6/52
Assessment
EPDS PHQ9
Score >12
Score <12
Review as necessary
Support
Accepted
Rejected
Literature
Websites
Apps
Contact Follow Up 2/52
Management Options
PC = Primary Care – PMH (Perinatal Mental Health)
Specialist service MW/HV/GP/Peer Support worker
SC = Secondary Care – MBU (Mother and Baby Unit)
SS = Social Service
NGO = Non Government Organisation/Charitable Organisations
AN = Antenatal
BV = Birth Visit
6/52 = 6 Weeks Post Delivery
EPDS = Edinburgh Postnatal Depression Scale
PHQ-9 = Patient Health Questionnaire 9
Copyright © Perinatal MH Training CIC 2023 All Rights Reserved

FIGURE 5.1

Other assessment tools

Other assessment tools are available, and some practitioners may prefer to use the Whooley Questions (Whooley *et al.*, 1997). They are straightforward and brief to answer, which can be useful for a busy practitioner. The two questions, each requiring a simple yes or no answer, ask:

1. 'During the past month, have you often been bothered by feeling down, depressed or hopeless?'
2. 'During the past month, have you often been bothered by little interest or pleasure in doing things?'

If the respondent answers yes to either of these questions, a follow-up question asks: 'Is this something you feel you need or want help with?'

The questions list core depressive symptoms stated in the *Diagnostic and Statistical Manual of Mental Disorders* (DSM-5: American Psychiatric Association, 2013), a clinical text that outlines the signs and symptoms of depression and other mental health conditions.

THERAPEUTIC INTERVENTIONS

Following the assessment of a parent, there are many possible routes to supporting their needs. Support can involve taking a holistic approach, exploring a parent's daily routines, interactions with their infant, exercise regime, employment, lifestyle choices, diet and alcohol intake, social experiences, domestic issues, and other factors that can affect mental health. Some parents may find medication helpful, while others may prefer to be referred to a support group or a specialised perinatal mental health service offering tailored interventions.

There are many forms of therapeutic interventions available, ranging from person-centred counselling and art and music therapy to cognitive behavioural techniques. Some of these services are available on the NHS, others are provided privately; it largely depends on the area and accessibility. Prior to commencing any therapy, it is wise for the parent to discuss the options with a GP or a specialist perinatal mental health specialist team to ensure the right intervention is chosen for the right reason. It is, however, not a pick-and-choose situation, but through careful discussion, the parent might reach the decision to access the type of intervention that is right for them.

The value of listening

For parents, being asked questions and knowing that a practitioner is listening can be cathartic. *'If you don't ask the question, then who will? And if you can't sort it, then who can?'* can be a useful mantra when working with families during the perinatal period.

The success of listening depends on the skill of being able to listen actively, typically during a one-hour session. In some cases, if the practitioner has been trained in and feels competent to carry out 'Listening Visits', sessions may take place for up to six weeks. Once a practitioner has supported parents to identify their main issues, the parents realise that the solution is not as difficult as they initially believed. Listening allows the opportunity for one-to-one contact, honesty and openness. It is an effective way of allowing parents the space and time to consolidate their own thoughts and understand the difference between a thought and a feeling. It is important that parents do not feel judged by the practitioner or that their sessions and conversations are not interrupted. This allows a non-judgemental approach. The focus is on the parent and to point out their strengths, capabilities and competencies. This can empower the parent to make their own lifestyle choices. Sometimes a journal is useful to keep track of the lifestyle changes that may occur during the period (Hanley, 2015).

Support groups

Effective support groups have a vision for the future, ideal goals and objectives. Partnerships are sometimes necessary as support systems need to be in place with the appropriate mental health services. The mental health of the organisers and facilitators should be considered with sessions for debriefing and clinical supervision. Safeguarding policies must be in place, particularly if the parents' infants are invited as part of the group. For a group to be successful, every member should have the opportunity to participate. Confidentiality should be observed and respected, listening encouraged, and rewards and failures shared. The group's agreed philosophy must always be kept in mind. For social media groups, it is also essential to ensure the trust and safety of the group and to be mindful of the vulnerability of some of the members. Support groups may be recommended by the health practitioner, by word of mouth or online.

Active support groups

Effective active groups include walking and talking groups, in which participants discuss their lives and issues while walking in green spaces. There are more and more different ways in which people are being encouraged to engage with the natural environment, for example, wild swimming and cold-immersion therapy sessions, which are proving to be increasingly popular. The camaraderie and team spirit of sport can also have therapeutic value; for example, participants can play football together and meet socially afterwards (Hendel, 2018).

Psychological interventions

Psychotherapy

Psychotherapy is a talking therapy that can help parents during the perinatal period. Interventions can enable parents to freely discuss their problems and therapists can pinpoint subjects or situations that may make parents feel uncomfortable, distressed or out of control. Discussing situations in depth can help parents understand why they feel as they do and discover how they can solve their problems by changing the way they think, which can, in turn, alter the way they feel. Psychotherapy can be the first line of treatment in perinatal depression because it is usually effective for between six months and a year following a depressive episode. One study found that the effects of psychotherapy on depression were moderate to large, with a positive secondary effect on anxiety, social support, parental and marital stress (Cuijpers *et al.*, 2021).

Person-centred therapy

As the name of this therapeutic approach suggests, it is centred around the person (or parent) and can encourage the desire and the capacity for personal growth and change. It is a form of psychotherapy that encourages and supports individuals to find solutions from within themselves.

Mentalisation-based therapy

This long-term therapeutic approach is useful for parents in difficult relationships or who have experienced intense emotional distress and overwhelming feelings. These feelings may have resulted in self-harm or aggression towards others. The therapy improves the parent's capacity to mentalise by focusing on what is happening in their mind and those of others, and to link this to understanding and alleviating problematic behaviours.

Solution-focused brief therapy

This is a series of three or four short sessions designed to promote positive change for a parent rather than prompting them to reflect on past problems. The parent is encouraged to set goals, work out how to achieve them, and then positively focus on what is done well.

Behavioural therapy

This form of therapy can be successful for parents who suffer from compulsive obsessive behaviours, phobias or addictions. It is based on the belief that unwanted or unhealthy behaviours are a learned response to past experiences, and it focuses on current problems. Its aim is to help parents to learn new, more positive behaviours without having to analyse the past.

Cognitive behavioural therapy (CBT)

This is one of the more popular forms of therapy for anxiety, depression, stress, phobias and eating disorders, and for managing long-term conditions. Its cognitive emphasis can help parents to change the way they think and enable them to behave differently rather than focusing on events that may have caused negative emotions. CBT can support parents to focus their thoughts on what is happening currently and offers practical solutions to help parents reorganise their thoughts, feelings and behaviour.

Mindfulness

Mindfulness is a simple, effective way to help deal with stress, anxiety, low self-worth and worry, among other mental health issues. It involves concentrating on the here and now, accepting what happens and focusing on it until it passes. It takes practice, but practitioners can guide parents through simple exercises (see Worksheet 7: Mindfulness). Mindfulness can be effective when a parent feels they are having moments of despair or losing control. Practising how to still the mind and concentrate on their surroundings can help parents feel relaxed.

Many online courses can teach parents mindfulness techniques, but practitioners can introduce the practice to help parents understand why it can be effective and refer parents to local mindfulness groups.

Family and relationship therapy

This therapeutic approach explores the family as a system and examines the relationships and dynamics between parents and children, rather than treating them individually. It allows all family members to express and investigate difficult thoughts and emotions they may be experiencing and can enable family members to understand

and appreciate how and why that person may be feeling as they do. The family can make changes within their relationships and their lifestyles, providing a platform to rebuild or strengthen existing relationships.

Creative therapies

Art therapy

This uses the creative process of making art to explore and communicate issues, feelings and emotions that some parents may find too difficult or distressing to express in words. It creates a safe place to draw, paint or do photography and modelling. It can be used with a parent or in a group, where everyone's input is shared. It is powerful in relieving stress and improving mental wellbeing. It is carried out by a qualified art therapist.

Other creative therapies

This involves a wide range of techniques that can help parents who find it difficult to express themselves verbally. It can take many forms: writing, dance and movement therapy, drama therapy and music therapy, all of which are designed to help the parent to communicate their feelings and emotions through those media.

Music therapy and music-based activities

Several studies around the world (some of them relating to the antenatal period) have highlighted the importance of music for parental wellbeing during the perinatal period (Nwebube, Glover & Stewart, 2017). Listening to music either alone or in a group has been found to be helpful in reducing anxiety and stress during the perinatal period. Some interventions have been designed for listening to music at home for mothers who are unable to attend group sessions.

In structured music groups, parents can learn how to use music to reduce anxiety and the symptoms of postnatal depression. The aim is to create a socially supportive network and enhance parents' mood. A traditional lullaby may be chosen, and the group are encouraged to add their own repertories. If required, the lyrics could be altered to draw on themes of resilience, the importance of social support and strategies that would help them to cope with their psychological or physical challenges (Friedman *et al.*, 2010; Sanfilippo, Stewart & Glover, 2021). Support groups may be available which offer this type of intervention; but if there is not, this might be a consideration for the practitioner to start up one.

'Music therapy' can only be carried out by a qualified music therapist, but listening to music with other people, or participating in a choir or with a group of musicians provides the enjoyment that can be shared with everyone.

Lullabies

Singing lullabies is a simple remedy that may help a parent to placate both their infant and themselves. Using lullabies to soothe a troubled infant is not as common as it used to be (Robertson, 2024), but it is an easy way to express feelings and emotions, sometimes without the use of words. It is possible for the parent to attune their singing to their infant's needs by acknowledging the infant's distress with empathetic movements. The rhythm of a lullaby helps a parent to gently rock their infant, helping to soothe and calm them, whereas a more robust sway can help an infant to understand that their parent acknowledges their distress. The natural, naive voice of a parent and the simplicity of the words in a lullaby can let an infant know they are safe and secure (Fancourt & Perkins, 2018; Hanley, 2010). As the popularity of lullabies has waned, practitioners can suggest that parents sing songs they are familiar with instead, bearing in mind that upbeat rhythms may not be so suitable.

Some studies have highlighted the contribution of professional musicians who work with families to create and sing lullabies that are personal to them and their infant (Nwebube *et al.*, 2017; Sanfilippo *et al.*, 2019). The mothers in these studies were encouraged to compose music and write lyrics, considering their own identity and the ways in which they nurture their infant. Understanding and harnessing the value of the music provided many areas in which the development of the infant could be supported. It has also been found that the social engagement involved in this work supported mothers' wellbeing, making them feel less anxious and more relaxed (Sanfilippo *et al.*, 2019).

General support strategies

Often, practitioners may not be trained to offer parents a specialised form of therapy; however, they may be able to refer parents to a perinatal mental health service. As waiting times for specialist services can be long, practitioners may want to try different approaches to supporting parents in the interim. Techniques can be used that are neither psychotherapeutic nor invasive but may help parents until they can access interventions.

Breathing

Teaching anxious parents how to manage their breathing is important as it lowers blood pressure and heart rate, reduces stress hormones in the blood and lactic acid build-up in the tissues, balances the levels of oxygen and carbon dioxide in the blood, and increases feelings of calm and wellbeing. When a parent is under stress, their breathing pattern changes. When a parent is anxious, they may take short shallow breaths, using their shoulders rather than the diaphragm to move the air in and out of the lungs. This causes a disruption of the gases in the bloodstream. Shallow over-breathing or hyperventilation can prolong feelings of anxiety by increasing the physical symptoms of stress.

Practitioners can help parents to deliberately change and control the rhythm of their breathing by suggesting that they find a comfortable place to sit and then breathe in for a count of three and out for a count of three. In this practice, air is exhaled through the mouth and as the air comes out, the lips should be pursed, and the jaws should be slightly relaxed. This technique is repeated until calmness supersedes anxiety. A parent can be encouraged to practice this technique any time they feel anxious.

Grounding

This is a way to learn to focus on the present moment, helping parents to feel calmer and to think more clearly. By holding on to something to keep steady and still, the idea is to encourage parents to imagine being rooted to the ground before counting down from five to one.

The practitioner can help parents to understand and use this simple technique when they feel overwhelmed or that their anxiety is increasing.

Case study: Maya and David's experiences of therapy

Maya had suffered from birth trauma and had previous episodes of depression. She attended clinic with her infant son and, after completing an assessment form, became distressed. It appeared that Maya was not enjoying motherhood, found it difficult to sleep, had intrusive thoughts, blamed herself for everything that went wrong and said she had difficulty bonding with her son. Maya said the relationship with her husband, David, was tough, and they had not been intimate since she was pregnant. She said that their cultural values and gender-role differences had created pressures from family and friends for them to behave in a certain manner, and they were mindful of these expectations. Maya felt overwhelmed with her feelings of anxiety, and her husband was finding it difficult to manage Maya's wellbeing.

The practitioner listened to Maya's story and offered to teach her some mindfulness and breathing techniques to help lower her anxiety. However, although Maya found them helpful, she continued to be plagued by intrusive thoughts and had trouble sleeping. Maya and her husband were referred to a perinatal mental health psychologist.

When they first saw the psychologist, they found it difficult to let go of their distinct understandings of the birth trauma they experienced and the stress of the 'deontic operators' they encountered: the 'shoulds' and 'musts' they heard from professionals and relatives.

They both thought that professionals were 'telling' them what they should be feeling and not empathising with how they felt as new parents. Although David was always there for Maya and was happy to take on his commitment and responsibilities, he found that during the initial period following the birth, he too lacked support.

As their therapy continued, David and Maya found they were able to trust the process and began to support each other better. They both learned what triggered their anxieties and looked in depth at how these subtly overwhelmed them. Learning several coping strategies, they both discovered ways of managing their thoughts and feelings. Maya and David managed to challenge the expectations of how new parents ought to do things and how they should raise their child. After six months of therapy, they both felt that they were in a more stable and harmonious relationship.

Reflection points:

- What culturally sensitive knowledge points would practitioners need to support Maya and David?
- What would indicate that David needed support too?

Providing culturally sensitive support

There have been significant changes within the health and social care system to ensure that practitioners are culturally competent and sensitive, enabling them to address the needs of parents from ethnic minorities. There may be different needs between those who have been in the UK for generations and those who have recently arrived, such as asylum seekers or migrants.

In some studies, many mothers from ethnic minorities felt that they had not received the services they really needed (MacLellan *et al.*, 2022; Toh & Shorey, 2022). They reported suffering in silence because they did not feel confident to share how they felt and they sensed that the attitude of the practitioners was that they did not listen and did not care, emphasising ingrained racial prejudice. Criticism has been focused on the way antenatal care appears to be differently provided for white and black mothers. There are many challenges for providers that have been blamed on structural racism within the healthcare system.

Several studies have discussed the disproportionately high number of negative outcomes for mothers from ethnic minorities. To tackle systemic racism, there must be an understanding of the many forms of racial discrimination and embedded prejudices to learn how injustices can affect the care of parents.

Cultural competency refers to the ability of practitioners to provide and adapt to the needs of parents with diverse values, beliefs and behaviours. It is vital for practitioners to acquaint themselves with the culture of the parent and if the parents were born in this country, how their cultural nuances impact on their family life and support them in their child rearing practices and their emotional wellbeing. The cultural, social and language needs of parents who have recently arrived in the country should be considered and addressed to ensure care and support is tailored to their needs.

Where English is not the parents' first language, care should be provided by someone who can speak in the parent's own language or translation services should be used. Practitioners must listen to all parents' stories and try to understand that somatic symptoms, which may include headaches or upset stomachs, might be indicative of a perinatal mental disorder. Good communication skills and cultural sensitivity are prerequisites when working with parents; practitioners should show compassion and not dismiss parents' fears or anxieties but takes the time to listen to them.

Effective communication by a practitioner with expertise in

perinatal mental health can help to foster community and parental awareness of the importance of good mental health during the perinatal period, as well as encouraging the expression of feelings of depression and anxiety. It can also help to develop trust within a community and to establish a rapport with the parents. Once this is established, other parents may feel confident to come forward and share their lived experiences. This can culminate in the formation of support groups to sustain the mental wellbeing of the community and ultimately the individual parent.

Case study: Yasmin's experiences as an asylum seeker

Yasmin had made the treacherous journey to the UK. It took her over six months, but she felt it was worth it as she had wanted to join her husband, to have a better life. As a political dissident, her husband had been subjected to torture from government officials in their country. He was able to escape and enter the UK as an asylum seeker.

Several months after arriving, Yasmin became pregnant. Yasmin could not get used to the racial abuse she suffered. She had heard that the UK was a good country with good values and was bitterly disappointed with the treatment she received from some people. Her husband was unable to work, and they had to live in temporary accommodation. Yasmin was not used to the cold. Their heating system was old, and black mould grew on the walls. Yasmin delivered a baby boy. Yasmin missed her mother who lived back in her home country and felt she should not bother the services.

A health practitioner called to examine the infant and noticed Yasmin's distress. Although Yasmin spoke little English, the health practitioner was able to establish that Yasmin's mood was low as she looked sad, avoided eye contact, and the tone of her voice was flat. The practitioner realised that Yasmin needed to see her doctor and agreed with her to make a GP appointment. The health practitioner also considered Yasmin's cultural and religious background and recommended a community group for Muslim women in the local area. With support from healthcare services Yasmin was able to access both medication and culturally supportive care.

Reflection points:

- How could practitioners have identified that Yasmin was at risk of perinatal illness?
- What support strategies could a practitioner implement?

MEDICATION

There are instances when the use of medication may be indicated because the parent is suffering from anxiety or depression. A parent may be so preoccupied with their thoughts and feelings that they are unable to concentrate on words and procedures, which may hamper any therapeutic work.

Medication is always prescribed by a clinician who monitors a parent's side-effects and responses. Contrary to popular belief, much modern medication for mental health conditions is well tolerated and the side-effects, if any are present, are usually mild. Antidepressant medication usually starts to be effective two to three weeks after it is first taken and should normally be taken for at least six to nine months, depending on clinical advice. Some antidepressants are SSRIs (selective serotonin reuptake inhibitors) and are very effective in the treatment of depression.

It can be helpful for practitioners to have an awareness of the side-effects of medications used to improve perinatal mental health conditions so they can effectively reassure and support parents. Some parents taking medication may notice an increase in their appetite and, as a consequence, experience unwanted weight gain. However, sometimes it is difficult to ascertain whether the antidepressants are associated with weight gain or if it is caused by lifestyle choices. Sometimes, weight gain may occur because depression reduces and the appetite improves.

Parents taking antidepressant medication may also experience a loss of sexual desire or a change in their desire for sex, problems with arousal, erectile dysfunction, discomfort, dissatisfaction and or decreased orgasms. The severity of sexual side-effects, if they are experienced, depends on the individual and the specific type and dose of the antidepressant.

SUMMARY

Numerous methods and techniques can be used to support parents, but the suitability of the practice or therapy is important. As with any management or treatment, it requires the support, skills and knowledge of the practitioner to guide parents towards the best possible options for them. When a parent's mind is at peace, it is more active and rational, enabling greater focus and more effective problem-solving and decision-making. This clarity of mind can help parents to find positive solutions to the challenges they face, and it allows the synergy of the mind and body, enhancing perinatal mental health and emotional wellbeing.

USEFUL RESOURCES

Art therapy

British Association of Art Therapists: https://baat.org

Music therapy

British Association for Music Therapy: www.bamt.org

Assessment forms

PHQ-9 Depression Test Questionnaire: https://patient.info/doctor/patient-health-questionnaire-phq-9

Hanwill Model of Assessment (see Figure 5.1)

Counselling and psychotherapy

The British Association for Counselling and Psychotherapy (BACP) is the professional association for members of the counselling professions in the UK. Its members offers solution-focused therapy, mentalisation therapy, behavioural therapy, CBT and family therapy: www.bacp.co.uk

Mindfulness

Headspace is a calming mindfulness app: www.headspace.com

Breathworks provides mindfulness training for NHS staff: www.breathworks-mindfulness.org.uk/nhs-mindfulness-training-for-health-professionals

CHAPTER-SPECIFIC WORKSHEETS FOR PRACTITIONERS (SEE APPENDIX)

Worksheet 2: Supporting fathers in the antenatal period

Worksheet 5: Lifestyle choices in the perinatal period

Worksheet 7: Mindfulness

Worksheet 8: Thoughts, feelings and behaviours

CHAPTER 6

Reflections

Parenthood can be joyous and fulfilling, enabling parents to experience and develop new roles and identities. However, it can also be intense and overwhelming, and mental health conditions affecting both mothers and fathers are common in the perinatal period.

Difficulties during the perinatal period can affect lifestyle choices. Pregnancies can be stressful, causing severe anxiety that may have consequences for the parent and the unborn infant. Once an infant is born, the lives of new parents often change significantly.

Allowing parents to talk openly about how they feel during this transformative time can be cathartic. Practitioners can encourage honest conversations about parents' experiences, supporting them to manage challenges, make the most of opportunities, and improve their lifestyles. Factors that can improve parents' general wellbeing include socialising with family and friends, adopting a healthy diet, limiting or stopping the consumption of alcohol and recreational drugs, exercising and sleeping well.

COMPASSION FATIGUE

Practitioners will be familiar with the benefits that a compassionate approach can bring to parents. However, it is important to be conscious that caring work can be emotionally demanding; the toll on practitioners' mental health can be difficult to recognise as they are required to manage or suppress their own feelings in a professional context. Compassion can quickly develop into fatigue, which can be mentally and physically exhausting. Practitioners can become preoccupied with parents' pain, ruminating over their problems at the expense of their own wellbeing. If they are not managed, these feelings can evolve into intrusive thoughts, irritability, avoidance and sleep problems. These symptoms may undermine a practitioner's confidence, increase their anxiety and decrease their capacity to work, leading to negative coping behaviours.

These challenging feelings may affect practitioners' leisure and family time, damaging relationships and negatively impacting mental health (Cocker & Joss, 2016). Compassion fatigue mimics a form of secondary traumatic stress and 'burnout', which can happen as a consequence of over-exposure to other people's distressing experiences. Acknowledging that there is a problem and recognising the steady erosion of work–life balance is the first step to supporting recovery in this situation. Support from colleagues is vital, as is effective management and the provision of useful resources, supervision and positive feedback.

SUPPORTING PARENTS AND INFANTS TO THRIVE

To effectively support parents during the perinatal period, practitioners need a strong knowledge base, excellent listening skills, and an empathetic awareness of the pitfalls and privileges of early parenthood. This provides solid foundations for practitioners to do the valuable job of helping parents to prepare for challenges that they may encounter. A supportive professional context will enable practitioners to best understand how parents feel and how to help them. No parent should suffer in silence with the symptoms of mental health conditions, and practitioners can contribute to equipping parents in their care with the skills and resources to maintain and develop wellbeing and resilience. All infants deserve the best possible start in life, and all parents deserve the opportunity to enjoy the transformative experience of becoming and being a parent.

CHAPTER-SPECIFIC WORKSHEETS FOR PRACTITIONERS (SEE APPENDIX)

Worksheet 10: A reflective diary for practitioners

APPENDIX

Worksheets

Worksheets in the appendix are downloadable from https://www.jkp.com/catalogue/book/9781839970375.

WORKSHEET 1

PREGNANCY

Practitioners can use this worksheet to ask parents about their overall feelings relating to their pregnancy.

1. How do you feel about the pregnancy?

   ☺ .... ☹

2. Do you know why you feel like this?

   ☺ .... ☹

What about writing down your feelings ?

I feel ....

Exhausted

Elated

Nervous

Angry

Irritated

Excited

Can you understand why you feel like this?

☺ .... ☹

If you have difficult feelings about the pregnancy, how do you cope?

For example:

- Talk?...... With partner/midwife/mother/father/friends/family
- Drink lots of coffee
- Consume more than your usual amount of alcohol
- Gamble ?...... Casino/online/on phone
- Nothing?

- ....
- ....
- ....
- ....

Do you feel you need greater support?

....

....

....

....

Do you know where you can seek help?

....

....

....

....

WORKSHEET 2

SUPPORTING FATHERS IN THE ANTENATAL PERIOD

Practitioners can use this worksheet to involve fathers from the start of the antenatal period. It is aimed at fathers who may find it difficult to ask the right questions and feel they need further information. Sometimes, fathers cannot make the antenatal clinic appointments, so this worksheet provides helpful hints on how to manage this

Helpful hints for fathers

If you are unable to attend antenatal appointments or appointments with doctors:

- Can you make an appointment to join via Zoom or video call?
- What about WhatsApp or FaceTime?

Many midwives now provide a list of questions and answers to inform the father about the progress of the pregnancy, but if this is not available then it is advisable to compose a checklist of questions that can be given to the midwife.

What will you be asking to make life easier for the mother?

....

....

....

....

How can you help the mother during the pregnancy?

....

....

....

....

How can you be more prepared for parenthood?

....

....

....

....

Here are some examples of things you may want to find out about:

1. What foods should be avoided?
2. What is the advice about alcohol?
3. How much rest should the mother have?
4. What can I do at this stage do engage with my baby?
5. How can I engage with my baby?
6. What can I do to make life less stressful for the mother?
7. What responsibilities can I take on to help the mother during her pregnancy?

THE PERINATAL PERIOD

Practitioners might want to ask parents the following questions during the postnatal period.

- How did you feel about the pregnancy?
- Did things go according to plan?
- In what way have things changed since the infant's birth?
- Are you aware that both parents can experience low mood after the baby is born?

If the father or partner is unable to attend the clinic and cannot join via Zoom, WhatsApp or FaceTime, then the following list of questions could be considered. The mother can give the list to her partner so they can tick off the questions they would like answers to.

Questions

It is important to share any concerns you may have with a practitioner. There is no such thing as a stupid question:

- How much rest should my partner have?
- How can I reduce our stress?
- What can I do to engage with my infant?
- How can I contact you if I have any further concerns or questions?
- How many clinic appointments are there, and how many can I attend?
- If I feel I need to talk with someone, who should I contact?
- Are there any specialist perinatal mental health teams and will I be able to contact them?

WORKSHEET 4

THINKING ABOUT OLDER CHILDREN

Practitioners can use this worksheet to ask parents about their older children.

- How are your other children doing?
- How are they getting on at school?
- How are their friendships with other children?
- How do they feel about you being unwell?
- Do you know if they are worried about anything?
- Has their behaviour changed and, if so, how?
- It there anyone there to support them when you are feeling unwell?

LIFESTYLE CHOICES IN THE PERINATAL PERIOD

Practitioners can use this worksheet to ask parents about their lifestyle choices and enquire about whether they have any anxieties.

Questions for parents-to-be
Please take a moment to consider your lifestyle.

Please fill in each question about how you feel on a scale 0–10 (0 is 'not applicable', 1 is 'not good', 10 is 'very good'). Please explain your answer.

- How would you rate your diet?

  ....

  ....

- What do you feel about your alcohol intake?

  ....

  ....

- What do you feel about your sleep pattern?

  ....

  ....

- How do you feel about any substances you take?

  ....

  ....

- Have you or someone else been affected by gambling harms?

  ....

  ....

- How active are you?

  ....

  ....

Please take a moment to consider any stressors you may have.

- Can you list things that make you feel stressed?

  ....

  ....

- Can you list things that make you feel low?

  ....

  ....

Do you know how long these stressors have been a problem?

....

....

Are they manageable?

....

....

A reflective activity about support networks

- Draw a large circle in the centre of a piece of paper and write your name inside it.
- On the outside, write down all the people that currently support you and put an arrow towards your name. The thicker the arrow the more support they offer you.
- Circle the names of the people who make you feel good.
- Examining the chart, how does it make you feel, and what changes would you like to make?

WORKSHEET 6

INTERACTIONS BETWEEN MOOD AND LIFESTYLE

Practitioners can use this worksheet with parents to help them to understand how their mood affects their lifestyle and vice versa.

Daily mood rating form

Please rate your mood for each day over a two-week period using the ten-point scale shown. A low number means that you felt bad and a high number means that you felt good:

Very depressed......................................Very happy

1 2 3 4 5 6 7 8 9 10

Mood Score (starting date ....)

Day	Date	Mood Score
1		
2		
3		
4		
5		
6		
7		
8		
9		
10		
11		
12		
13		
14		

What causes you the most stress?

For example:

- Mealtimes
- Getting ready to go to work
- Bedtime
- Changes in routine
- Shopping
- Working late

- ....
- ....
- ....
- ....

What are the early signs that you are becoming stressed?

For example:

- Shouting more than usual
- Clenching teeth
- Having palpitations
- Experiencing unexplained pains
- Feeling overwhelmed

- ....
- ....
- ....
- ....

List the kinds of activities which you find pleasant:

For example:

- Going for a walk
- Meeting up with friends
- Enjoying a long soak in the bath
- Listening to music
- Going out for a meal
- Having a haircut
- Paying a compliment

- ....
- ....
- ....
- ....

Please list your top ten favourite activities

1. ....
2. ....
3. ....
4. ....
5. ....
6. ....
7. ....
8. ....
9. ....
10. ....

Now consider which activities you manage to do on a regular basis and which activities you do not manage to do on a regular basis. How does that make you feel?

....

....

....

....

....

WORKSHEET 7

MINDFULNESS

Practitioners can use this worksheet to support parents to feel present in the moment. It can be carried out doing nothing or whilst doing a task.

Exercise 1

Ask the parent to sit quietly, preferably in an open space, and take a deep breath, then ask the following questions:

- What can you see? Look at the objects in the room or, if you are outside, look at the sky and the clouds. What are the shapes? What are the colours?
- What can you feel? What is the sensation you have sitting down? What does the ground beneath your feet feel like? Is there a breeze or a fan heater blowing against your face?
- What can you hear? Is there a buzz of machinery in the background? Are birds singing? Can you hear people chatting?
- What can you smell? The smell of newly cut grass, freshly made coffee, or someone's perfume perhaps?
- Focus on yourself: How does your body feel? Are you warm? Are you cold? Do you feel relaxed?
- Focus on your breathing.
- How did that make you feel?

Exercise 2

This is an exercise you can share with the parent so they can learn to feel present while doing a task. They can achieve a relaxing, meditative state by listening to their senses. A good example of a time to try this exercise is while brushing teeth: how often do we think about the movement of the brush, the taste of the toothpaste and which teeth are being brushed? Housework will be another familiar repetitive occupation for parents that is often done automatically while ruminating over other thoughts. The process of the actual job can be overlooked.

For example, when washing dishes:

- What can you see? (e.g. What colour is the crockery? What is it made of? How many pieces can you count? What foodstuffs need to be washed off? What else can you see?)

- What can you feel? (e.g. What is the temperature of the water? Does the water feel hard or soft? What is the sensation while you are standing at the sink?)

- What can you hear? (e.g. Is the water running fast or slow? What can be heard in the distance?)

- What can you smell? (e.g. What does the washing-up liquid smell of? Are there any other scents in the room?)

- Focus on yourself: How does your body feel? Are you warm? Are you cold? Do you feel relaxed?

- Focus on your breathing.

- How did that make you feel?

For example, rocking your infant to sleep:

- What can you see? (e.g. What is your infant wearing? What colours are their clothes? What else is in the room?)
- What can you feel? (e.g. Can you feel the warmth of your infant? Is there a gentle breeze? Can you feel the infant's weight in your arms?)
- What can you hear? (e.g. Can you hear your infant's breathing? Can you hear your infant's sounds? What other sounds are around you?)
- What can you smell? (e.g. Can you smell the infant's body? Can you smell freshly laundered clothes? Are there other smells in the room?)
- Focus on yourself: How does your body feel? Are you warm? Are you cold? Do you feel relaxed?
- Focus on your breathing.
- How did that make you feel?

WORKSHEET 8

THOUGHTS, FEELINGS AND BEHAVIOURS

Practitioners can use this worksheet with parents to help them understand the difference between their thoughts and feelings.

Often, our thoughts and feelings are confused. We can think negatively which makes us feel negative and, therefore, behave negatively. Changing the way you think is not easy, particularly if you are anxious or feel depressed. However, trying to think positively will make you feel positive and behave positively.

A **thought** is the process of using the mind to think about an idea or something similar. For example: *I think I am a bad parent because my sister can settle my son without any trouble, and he cries even more when I try to settle him. I am not as good a parent as my sister.*

A **feeling** is an emotion, such as anger or happiness. For example: *I feel frustrated because my sister is better at settling my son but also hopeless because I am unable to do it.*

A **behaviour** is how you react. For example: *I will let my sister settle my baby as she is better at it than I am or I will ask my sister for advice.*

Try to think of positive examples, such as.

- I really am a pretty good mother.
- That makes me feel okay, I feel happy about myself.
- I smile and cuddle my baby, and she loves it!

Now think about the statements in the table below and write your answers in the next column – deciding what is a thought, what is a feeling and how that makes you behave.

Statements	**What are your thoughts?**	**How does that make you feel?**	**How do you think you behave when you feel this way?**
EXAMPLE What does being a parent mean to you?	*I am glad I have the opportunity.*	*I feel happy and excited.*	*I want to show off my son to everyone.*
What does being a parent mean to you?			

WORKSHEET 9

PARTNER SUPPORT

A parent's mental health can improve significantly if they have consistent support from their partner. Here are some points that a practitioner might like to discuss with the partner to help them understand how to be supportive.

- Partners can make a marked difference to wellbeing.
- Mental health conditions must be taken seriously.
- Denying your partner's depression can make the recovery process longer.
- The more that is expected of your partner, the longer the recovery process.

The partner may have worries about saying the wrong thing and may feel that:

- Any attempt to try to say the right thing may be met with contempt.
- If they say they love their partner, they may not be believed.
- If they tell their partner they are a good parent, they may feel they are being patronised.
- If they tell them not to worry, they will 'know' they do not have any idea about how they are feeling.
- If they tell them they should return to work early, they will feel guilty as they feel they should be working harder.

In fact, while anything that might be said will not be perfect, the important thing is that they care and are willing to offer support. Be aware and notice the kinds of things that can trigger anxiety and depression. Mind offers these tips to offer a way forward.[1]

1 © Mind. This information is published in full at mind.org.uk

Recommendations for offering emotional support:

- *Listen. Simply giving someone space to talk, and listening to how they're feeling, can be really helpful in itself. If they're finding it difficult, let them know that you're there when they are ready.*

- *Offer reassurance. Seeking help can feel lonely, and sometimes scary. You can reassure someone by letting them know that they are not alone, and that you will be there to help.*

- *Stay calm. Even though it might be upsetting to hear that someone you care about is distressed, try to stay calm. This will also help your friend or family member feel calmer and show them that they can talk to you openly without upsetting you.*

- *Be patient. You might want to know more details about their thoughts and feelings or want them to get help immediately. But it's important to let them set the pace for seeking support themselves.*

- *Try not to make assumptions. Your perspective might be useful to your friend or family member, but try not to assume that you already know what may have caused their feelings, or what will help.*

Mind also suggest that keeping social contact for the person who is having difficulty is important. This could mean making sure they are still involved in social events and making sure that things feel as normal as possible by still talking about other parts of their lives.

Practitioners should also advise on paths for emergency support for crisis situations.

WORKSHEET 10

A REFLECTIVE DIARY FOR PRACTITIONERS

Try to fill this in each week.

- How do you feel about your current lifestyle?
  - The positive things

    ....

    ....

  - The negative things

    ....

    ....

- What is your work–life balance like?
  - The positive things

    ....

    ....

  - The negative things

    ....

    ....

- Family life
  - What do you feel is good about your family life?

    ....

    ....

– What is bad about your family life?

....

....

- Friends
  - Who are you able to talk to?

....

....

  - How would they be able to help you?

....

....

TICK THE FEELINGS YOU HAVE EXPERIENCED OVER THE PAST WEEK

1	2	3	4	5	6
Happy	Relaxed	Able	Nervous	Unsure	Tearful
Inspired	Calm	Brave	Anxious	Confused	Angry
Hopeful	Content	Assertive	Cautious	Frustrated	Low
Pleased	Proud	Positive	Tired	Irritated	Unloved
Valued	Relieved	Confident	Troubled	Agitated	Cheerful

Make a list of people and organisations who can help you:

....

....

....

....

References

Aarestrup, A.K., Skovgaard Væver, M., Petersen, J., Røhder, K. & Schiøtz, M. (2020). An early intervention to promote maternal sensitivity in the perinatal period for women with psychosocial vulnerabilities: Study protocol of a randomized controlled trial. *BMC Psychology, 8*, 41. https://doi.org/10.1186/s40359-020-00407-3

Abraham, S. (2016.). *Eating Disorders: The Facts*. Oxford University Press.

Alder, J., Stadlmayr, W., Tschudin, S. & Bitzer, J. (2006). Post-traumatic symptoms after childbirth: What should we offer? *Journal of Psychosomatic Obstetrics & Gynecology, 27*(2), 107–112. https://doi.org/10.1080/01674820600714632

Alhusen, J.L., Ray, E., Sharps, P. & Bullock, L. (2015). Intimate partner violence during pregnancy: maternal and neonatal outcomes. *Journal of Women's Health, 24*(1), 100–106. https://doi.org/10.1089/jwh.2014.4872

Alptekin, F.B., Güngör, B.B., Öztürk, N. & Aydin, N. (2022). Mother–infant bonding in patients with bipolar disorder. *Archives of Neuropsychiatry, 59*, 183–187.

American Psychiatric Association (1994). *Diagnostic and Statistical Manual of Psychiatric Disorders* (4th edn: DSM-IV). American Psychiatric Publishing.

American Psychiatric Association (2013). *Diagnostic and Statistical Manual of Psychiatric Disorders* (5th edn: DSM-5). American Psychiatric Publishing.

Amjad, S., Chojecki, D., Osornio-Vargas A. & Ospina, M.B. (2021). Wildfire exposure during pregnancy and the risk of adverse birth outcomes: A systematic review. *Environment International, 156*. https://doi.org/10.1016/j.envint.2021.106644

Anke, T.M.S., Slinning, K., Moe, V., Brunborg, C. *et al.* (2020). Bipolar offspring and mothers: interactional challenges at infant age 3 and 12 months – a developmental pathway to enhanced risk? *International Journal of Bipolar Disorders, 8*, 27. https://doi.org/10.1186/s40345-020-00192-3

Auxéméry Y. (2018). Post-traumatic psychiatric disorders: PTSD is not the only diagnosis. *La Presse Médicale, 47*(5), 423–430. https://doi.org/10.1016/j.lpm.2017.12.006

Babenko, O., Kovalchuk, I. & Metz, G.A. (2015). Stress-induced perinatal and transgenerational epigenetic programming of brain development and mental health. *Neuroscience & Biobehavioral Reviews, 48*, 70–91. https://doi.org/10.1016/j.neubiorev.2014.11.013

Babetin, K. (2020). The birth of a mother: A psychological transformation. *Journal of Prenatal & Perinatal Psychology & Health, 34*(5), 410–428.

Ballard, C. & Davies, R. (1996). Postnatal depression in fathers. *International Review of Psychiatry, 8*(1), 65–71.

Barkham, M., Bewick, B., Mullin, T., Gilbody, S. *et al.* (2013). The CORE-10: A short measure of psychological distress for routine use in the psychological therapies. *Counselling and Psychotherapy Research, 13*(1), 3–13. http://doi.org/10.1080/14733145.2012.729069

Bastos, M.H., Furuta, M., Small, R., McKenzie-McHarg, K. & Bick, D. (2015). Debriefing interventions for the prevention of psychological trauma in women following childbirth. *Cochrane Database of Systematic Reviews,* Issue 4, CD007194. https://doi.org/10.1002/14651858.CD007194.pub2

Bastos, R.A., Campos, L.S., Faria-Schützer, D.B., Brito, M.E. *et al.* (2022). Offspring of mothers with bipolar disorder: A systematic review considering personality features. *Brazilian Journal of Psychiatry, 44*(1), 94–102. https://doi.org/10.1590/1516-4446-2020-1465

Bauer, A., Tinelli, M. & Knapp, M. (2022). *The economic case for increasing access to treatment for women with common mental health problems during the perinatal period.* Care Policy and Evaluation Centre London School of Economics and Political Science. https://www.researchgate.net/publication/359257318_The_economic_case_for_increasing_access_to_treatment_for_women_with_common_mental_health_problems_during_the_perinatal_period

BEAT Eating Disorders (n.d.). *Orthorexia.* https://www.beateatingdisorders.org.uk/get-information-and-support/about-eating-disorders/types/other-eating-feeding-problems/orthorexia/

Beck, C.T., Watson, S. & Gable, R. K. (2018). Traumatic childbirth and its aftermath: Is there anything positive? *Journal of Perinatal Education, 27*(3), 175–184.

Bergstrom, M. (2013). Depressive symptoms in new first-time fathers: Associations with age, sociodemographic characteristics, and antenatal psychological well-being. *Birth: Issues in Perinatal Care, 40*(1), 32–38. https//doi.org/10.1111/Birt.12026

Beversdorf, D.Q., Stevens, H.E., Margolis. K.G. & Van de Water, J. (2019). Prenatal stress and maternal immune dysregulation in autism spectrum disorders: Potential points for intervention. *Current Pharmaceutical Design, 25*(41), 4331–4343. https://doi.org/10.2174/1381612825666191119093335

Biaggi, A., Conroy, S., Pawlby, S. & Pariante, C.M. (2016). Identifying the women at risk of antenatal anxiety and depression: A systematic review. *Journal of Affective Disorders, 191*, 62–77. https://doi.org/10.1016/j.jad.2015.11.014

Boekhorst, M.G., Beerthuizen, A., Hillegers, M., Pop, V.J. & Bergink, V. (2021). Mother-to-infant bonding in women with a bipolar spectrum disorder. *Obstetric and Pediatric Pharmacology, 9*. https://doi.org/10.3389/fped.2021.646985

Borra, C., Iacovou, M. & Sevilla, A. (2015). new evidence on breastfeeding and postpartum depression: The importance of understanding women's intentions. *Maternal and Child Health Journal, 19*, 897–907. https://doi.org/10.1007/s10995-014-1591-z

Bozzatello, P., Rocca, P., Baldassarre, L., Bosia, M. & Bellino, S. (2021). The role of trauma in early onset borderline personality disorder: A biopsychosocial perspective. *Frontiers in Psychiatry, 12*, 721361. https://doi.org/10.3389/fpsyt.2021.721361

Brock, H., Rizvi, A. & Hany, M. (2025). Obsessive-compulsive disorder. [Updated 24 February 2024]. In *StatPearls* [Internet]. StatPearls Publishing. www.ncbi.nlm.nih.gov/books/NBK553162

Brown, A. & Davies, R. (2014). Fathers' experiences of supporting breastfeeding: Challenges for breastfeeding promotion and education. *Maternal & Child Nutrition 10*(4), 510–526. https://doi.org/10.1111/mcn.12129

Brown, A., Raynor, P. & Lee, M. (2011). Healthcare professionals' and mothers' perceptions of factors that influence decisions to breastfeed or formula feed infants: A comparative study. *Journal of Advanced Nursing, 67*(9), 1993–2003. https://doi.org/10.1111/j.1365-2648.2011.05647.x

Byrne, V., Egan, J., Mac Neela, P. & Sarma, K. (2017). What about me? The loss of self through the experience of traumatic childbirth, *Midwifery, 51*, 1–11. https://doi.org/10.1016/j.midw.2017.04.017

Cacciatore, J., Killian, M. & Harper, M. (2016). Adverse outcomes in bereaved mothers: The importance of household income and education. *SSM Population Health, 2*, 117–122. https://doi.org/10.1016/j.ssmph.2016.02.009

Campos-Garzón, C., Riquelme-Gallego, B., de la Torre-Luque, A. & Caparrós-González, R.A. (2021). Psychological impact of the COVID-19 pandemic on pregnant women: A scoping review. *Behavioral Sciences, 11*(12), 181. https://doi.org/10.3390/bs11120181

Carlberg, M., Edhborg, M. & Lindberg, L. (2018). Paternal perinatal depression assessed by the Edinburgh Postnatal Depression Scale and the Gotland Male Depression Scale: Prevalence and possible risk factors. *American Journal of Men's Health, 12*(4), 720–729. https://doi.org/10.1177/1557988317749071

Carlson, K., Mughal, S., Azhar, Y. & Siddiqui, W. (2022). Postnatal depression. In *StatPearls* [Internet]. StatPearls Publishing. www.ncbi.nlm.nih.gov/books/NBK519070

Chang, K.D., Blasey, C.M., Ketter, T.A. & Steiner, H. (2003). Temperament characteristics of child and adolescent bipolar offspring. *Journal of Affective Disorders, 77*(1), 11–19. https://doi.org/10.1016/s0165-0327(02)00105-2

Chapman, S.L. & Wu, L.T. (2013). Postpartum substance use and depressive symptoms: A review. *Women & Health, 53*(5), 479–503. https://doi.org/10.1080/03630242.2013.804025

Chen, K.W., Schultz, L. & Hughes, N. (2024). A case of postpartum obsessive-compulsive disorder in a first-time father, *Cureus, 16*(2), e54547. https://pmc.ncbi.nlm.nih.gov/articles/PMC10956711

Chin, K., Wendt, A., Bennett, I.M. & Bhat, A. (2022). Suicide and maternal mortality. *Current Psychiatry Reports, 24*(4), 239–275. https://doi.org/10.1007/s11920-022-01334-3

Coates, D., Davis, E. & Campbell, L. (2017). The experiences of women who have accessed a perinatal and infant mental health service: A qualitative investigation. *Advances in Mental Health, 15*(1), 88–100. https://doi.org/10.1007/s11920-022-01334-3

Cocker, F. & Joss, N. (2016). Compassion fatigue among healthcare, emergency and community service workers: A systematic review. *International Journal of Environmental Research and Public Health, 13*(6), 618. https://doi.org/10.3390/ijerph13060618

Collins, R. (2006). What is the purpose of debriefing women in the postnatal period? *Evidence-Based Midwifery*, 4(1).

Cooijmans, K.H.M., Beijers, R., Rovers, A.C. & de Weerth, C. (2017). Effectiveness of skin-to-skin contact versus care-as-usual in mothers and their full-term infants:

Study protocol for a parallel-group randomized controlled trial. *BMC Pediatrics, 17*(1), 154. https://doi.org/10.1186/s12887-017-0906-9

Cox, J. & Holden, J. (2003). *Perinatal Mental Health: A Guide to the Edinburgh Postnatal Depression Scale (EPDS)*. Royal College of Psychiatrists.

Cox, J., Holden, J. & Henshaw, C. (2014). *Perinatal Mental Health: The Edinburgh Postnatal Depression Scale (EPDS): Manual*. Royal College of Psychiatrists.

Cuijpers, P., Franco, P., Ciharova, M., Miguel, C. *et al.* (2021). Psychological treatment of perinatal depression: A meta-analysis. *Psychological Medicine, 53*(6), 2596–2608. https://doi.org/10.1017/S0033291721004529

Daniels, E., Arden-Close, E. & Mayers, A. (2020). Be quiet and man up: A qualitative questionnaire study into fathers who witnessed their partner's birth trauma. *BMC Pregnancy and Childbirth, 20*, 236. https://doi.org/10.1186/s12884-020-02902-2

Darwin, Z., Domoney, J., Iles, J., Bristow, F., McLeish, J., & Sethna, V. (2021). Involving and supporting partners and other family members in specialist perinatal mental health services: Good practice guide. NHS England. https://www.england.nhs.uk/wp-content/uploads/2021/03/Good-practice-guide-March-2021.pdf

Davies, W. (2017). Understanding the pathophysiology of postpartum psychosis: Challenges and new approaches. *World Journal of Psychiatry, 7*(2), 77–88. https://doi.org/10.5498/wjp.v7.i2.77

Deklava, L., Lubina, K., Circenis, K., Sudraba, V. & Millere, I. (2015). Causes of anxiety during pregnancy. *Procedia-Social and Behavioral Sciences, 205*, 623–626.

Dockrill, L. (2021). *What Have I Done: Motherhood, Mental Illness and Me*. Vintage.

Easey, K.E., Timpson, N. & Munafò, M.R. (2020). Association of prenatal alcohol exposure and offspring depression: A negative control analysis of maternal and partner consumption alcoholism. *Clinical and Experimental Research, 44*(5), 1132–1140. https://doi:10.1111/acer.14324

Edelstein, R.S., Wardecker, B.M., Chopik, W.J., Moors, A.C., Shipman, E.L. & Lin, N.J. (2014). Prenatal hormones in first-time expectant parents: Longitudinal changes and within-couple correlations *American Journal of Human Biology, 27*(3), 317–325. https://doi.org/10.1002/ajhb.22670

Elliott, J.K, Buchanan, K. & Bayes, S. (2024). The neurodivergent perinatal experience — A systematic literature review on autism and attention deficit hyperactivity disorder. *Women and Birth, 37*(6), 1871–5192. https://doi.org/10.1016/j.wombi.2024.101825

Erhuma, A.M. (2021). 'The Interaction between Maternal and Fetal Hypothalamic–Pituitary–Adrenal Axes.' In C. Pereira (Ed.). *Corticosteroids: A Paradigmatic Class Drug*. IntechOpen. www.intechopen.com/chapters/77382

Ertan, D., Hingray, C., Burlacu, E., Sterlé, A. & El-Hage, W. (2021). Post-traumatic stress disorder following childbirth. *BMC Psychiatry, 21*, 155. https://doi.org/10.1186/s12888-021-03158-6

Etheridge, J. & Slade, P. (2017). 'Nothing's actually happened to me.': The experiences of fathers who found childbirth traumatic. *BMC Pregnancy and Childbirth, 17*, 80. https://doi.org/10.1186/s12884-017-1259-y

Fairbrother, N., Collardeau, F., Albert, A., Challacombe, F.L. *et al.* (2021). High prevalence and incidence of obsessive-compulsive disorder among women across pregnancy and the postpartum. *Journal of Clinical Psychiatry, 82*(2), 20m13398. https://doi:10.4088/JCP.20m13398

Fancourt, D. & Perkins, R. (2018). The effects of mother–infant singing on emotional closeness, affect, anxiety, and stress hormones. *Music & Science, 1*. https://doi.org/10.1177/2059204317745746

Fogarty, A., McMahon, G., Findley, H., Hosking, C. *et al.* (2024). Prevalence of suicidal and self-harm ideation in fathers during the perinatal and early parenting period: A systematic review and meta-analysis. *Australian and New Zealand Journal of Psychiatry, 58*(12), 1020–1033. https//doi:10.1177/00048674241267896

Fried, L., Prohaska, T., Burholt, V., Burns, A. *et al.* (2020). A unified approach to loneliness. *Lancet 395*(10218), 114. https://doi.org/10.1016/S0140-6736(19)32533-4

Friedman, S., Kaplan, R., Rosenthal, M. & Console, P. (2010). Music therapy in perinatal psychiatry. *Music and Medicine, 2*, 219–225. https://doi.org/10.1177/1943862110379584

Gao X, Leng Y, Guo Y, Yang J. *et al.* (2019). Association between earthquake experience and depression 37 years after the Tangshan earthquake: A cross-sectional study. *BMJ Open, 9*(8), e026110. https://doi.org/10.1136/bmjopen-2018-026110

Gladstone, B., Boydell, K., Seeman, M. & McKeever, P. (2011). Children's experiences of parental mental illness: A literature review. *Early Intervention in Psychiatry, 5*, 271–289. doi.org/10.1111/j.1751-7893.2011.00287.x

Glover, V. (2014). Maternal depression, anxiety and stress during pregnancy and child outcome: What needs to be done. *Best Practice & Research. Clinical Obstetrics & Gynaecology, 28*(1), 25–35. https://doi.org/10.1016/j.bpobgyn.2013.08.017

Glover, V., O'Donnell, K., O'Connor, T. & Fisher, J. (2018). Prenatal maternal stress, fetal programming, and mechanisms underlying later psychopathology: A global perspective. *Development and Psychopathology, 30*(3), 843–854. https://doi.org/10.1017/S095457941800038X

Gobbi, G., Atkin, T., Zytynski, T., Wang, S. *et al.* (2019). Association of cannabis use in adolescence and risk of depression, anxiety, and suicidality in young adulthood: A systematic review and meta-analysis. *JAMA Psychiatry, 76*(4), 426–434. https://doi.org/10.1001/jamapsychiatry.2018.4500

Goldfarb, E.V. (2019). Enhancing memory with stress: Progress, challenges, and opportunities, *Brain and Cognition, 33*, 94–105. https://doi.org/10.1016/j.bandc.2018.11.009

Greenfield, M. & Darwin, Z. (2021). Trans and non-binary pregnancy, traumatic birth, and perinatal mental health: A scoping review. *International Journal of Transgender Health, 22*(1–2), 203–216. https://doi.org/10.1080/26895269.2020.1841057

Greenfield, M., Jomeen, J. & Glover, L. (2019). 'It can't be like last time': Choices made in early pregnancy by women who have previously experienced a traumatic birth. *Frontiers in Psychology, 10*, 56. https://doi.org/10.3389/fpsyg.2019.00056

Grizenko, N., Fortier, M.E., Zadorozny, C., Thakur, G. *et al.* (2012). Maternal stress during pregnancy, ADHD symptomatology in children and genotype: Gene-environment interaction. *Journal of the Canadian Academy of Child and Adolescent Psychiatry, 21*, 9–15.

Gross, D., Beeber, L., DeSocio, J. & Brennaman, L. (2016). Toxic stress: Urgent action needed to reduce exposure to toxic stress in pregnant women and young children. *Nursing Outlook, 64*, 513–515.

Gunn, J.K., Rosales, C.B., Center, K.E., Nuñez. A. *et al.* (2016). Prenatal exposure to cannabis and maternal and child health outcomes: A systematic review and meta-analysis. *BMJ Open. 6*(4), e009986. https://doi.org/10.1136/bmjopen-2015-009986

Gutierrez-Galve, L., Stein, A., Hanington, L., Heron, J. *et al.* (2019). Association of maternal and paternal depression in the postnatal period with offspring depression at age 18 years. *JAMA Psychiatry, 76*(3), 290–296. https://doi.org/10.1001/jamapsychiatry.2018.3667

Hambidge, S., Cowell, A., Arden-Close, E. & Mayers, A. (2021). 'What kind of man gets depressed after having a baby?' Fathers' experiences of mental health during the perinatal period. *BMC Pregnancy and Childbirth, 21*, 463. https://doi.org/10.1186/s12884-021-03947-7

Hanley, J. (2015). *Listening Visits in Perinatal Mental Health.* Routledge.

Hendel, H.J. (2018). *It's Not Always Depression: Working the Change Triangle to Listen to the Body, Discover Core Emotions and Connect to Your Authentic Self.* Random House.

Henshaw, C. (2000). Clinical and biological aspects of postpartum blues and depression. *Current Opinion in Psychiatry, 13*(6), 635–638.

Heron, J., O'Connor, T. G., Evans, J., Golding, J., Glover, V. & ALSPAC Study Team (2004). The course of anxiety and depression through pregnancy and the postpartum in a community sample. *Journal of Affective Disorders, 80*(1), 65–73.

Hofberg, K. & Brockington, I. (2000). Tokophobia: An unreasoning dread of childbirth: A series of 26 cases. *British Journal of Psychiatry, 176*(1), 83–85. https://doi.org/10.1192/bjp.176.1.83

Home Office (2019). Increase in crack cocaine use inquiry: Summary of findings. www.gov.uk/government/publications/crack-cocaine-increase-inquiry-findings/increase-in-crack-cocaine-use-inquiry-summary-of-findings

Honikman, J. (2022). *Postpartum Is Forever. Social Support from Conception through Grandparenthood.* Independently published. ISBN-13: 9798362779559

Howard, L., Poit, P. & Stein, A. (2014). No health without perinatal mental health. *The Lancet, 384*(9956), 1723–1724.

Howl, J. (2019). The perinatal dad engaging fathers in the perinatal period to support breastfeeding. www.fatherhoodinstitute.org/_files/ugd/efff1d_fbd7d19da9254aaf8c94c7a78eaf4721.pdf

Huang, X, Chen, L. & Zhang, L, (2019). Effects of paternal skin-to-skin contact in newborns and fathers after cesarean delivery. (2019). *Journal of Perinatal & Neonatal Nursing 33*(1), 68–73. https://doi.org/10.1097/JPN.0000000000000384

International Communicaffe (2021). *Seventy percent of Brits drink at least 2 cups of coffee per day, says survey.* https://www.comunicaffe.com/seventy-percent-of-brits-drink-at-least-2-cups-of-coffee-per-day-says-survey

Ionio, C., Ciuffo, G. & Landoni, M. (2021). Parent-infant skin-to-skin contact and stress regulation: A systematic review of the literature. *International Journal of Environmental Research and Public Health, 18*(9), 4695. https://doi.org/10.3390/ijerph18094695

Jones, I. & Craddock, N. (2005). Bipolar disorder and childbirth: The importance of recognising risk. *British Journal of Psychiatry, 186*(6), 453–454. https://doi.org/10.1192/bjp.186.6.453

Khalifeh, H., Hunt, I., Appleby, L. & Howard, L.M. (2016). Suicide in perinatal and non-perinatal women in contact with psychiatric services: 15-year findings from a UK national inquiry. *Lancet Psychiatry, 3*(3), 233–242. https://doi.org/10.1016/S2215-0366(16)00003-1

Kim, P. & Swain, J.E. (2007). Sad dads: Paternal postpartum depression. *Psychiatry (Edgmont), 4*(2), 35–47.

Kiviruusu, O. Pietikäinen, J.T., Kylliäinen, A., Pölkki, P. *et al.* (2020). Trajectories of mothers' and fathers' depressive symptoms from pregnancy to 24 months postpartum. *Journal of Affective Disorders, 260*, 629–637. https://doi.org/10.1016/j.jad.2019.09.038

Lancel, M., van Marle, H.J.F., Van Veen, M.M. & van Schagen, A.M. (2021). Disturbed sleep in PTSD: Thinking beyond nightmares. *Frontiers in Psychiatry, 12*, 767760. https://doi.org/10.3389/fpsyt.2021.767760

Lee, S.H., Liu, L.C., Kuo, P.C. & Lee, M.S. (2011). Postpartum depression and correlated factors in women who received in vitro fertilization treatment. *Journal of Midwifery and Women's Health, 56*(4), 347–352. https://doi.org/10.1111/j.1542-2011.2011.00033.x

Legazpi, P.C., Rodríguez-Muñoz, M., Le, H-N., Balbuena, C., Olivares, M.E. & Méndez, N.I. (2022). Suicidal ideation: Prevalence and risk factors during pregnancy. *Midwifery, 106*, 103226. https://doi.org/10.1016/j.midw.2021.103226

Letourneau, N., Leung, B., Ntanda, H., Dewey, D. *et al.* (2019). Maternal and paternal perinatal depressive symptoms associate with 2- and 3-year-old children's behaviour: Findings from the APrON longitudinal study. *BMC Pediatrics, 19*(1), 435. https://doi.org/10.1186/s12887-019-1775-1

Lindahl, V., Pearson, J. L. & Colpe, L. (2005). Prevalence of suicidality during pregnancy and the postpartum. *Archives of Women's Mental Health, 8*, 77–87.

MacLellan, J., Collins, S., Myatt, M., Pope, C., Knighton, W. & Rai, T. (2022). Black, Asian and minority ethnic women's experiences of maternity services in the UK: A qualitative evidence synthesis. *Journal of Advanced Nursing, 78*(7), 2175–2190. https://doi.org/10.1111/jan.15233

Mannion, C.A., Hobbs, A.J., McDonald, S.W. & Tough, S.C. (2013). Maternal perceptions of partner support during breastfeeding. *International Breastfeeding Journal, 8*, 4. https://doi.org/10.1186/1746-4358-8-4

Manthey, J., Freeman, T.P., Kilian, C., López-Pelayo, H. & Rehm, J. (2021). Public health monitoring of cannabis use in Europe: prevalence of use, cannabis potency, and treatment rates. *The Lancet Regional Health – Europe, 10*, 100227. https://doi.org/10.1016/j.lanepe.2021.100227

Matthey, S., Barnett., Kavanagh, D.J. & Howie, P. (2001). Validation of the Edinburgh Postnatal Depression Scale for men, and comparison of item endorsement with their partners. *Journal of Affective Disorders, 64*(2–3), 175–184. https://doi.org/10.1016/s0165-0327(00)00236-6

MBRRACE-UK (2020). *Saving Lives, Improving Mothers' Care: Lessons Learned To Inform Maternity Care from the UK and Ireland Confidential Enquiries into Maternal Deaths and Morbidity 2016–18.* www.npeu.ox.ac.uk/assets/downloads/mbrrace-uk/reports/maternal-report-2020/MBRRACE-UK_Maternal_Report_Dec_2020_v10_ONLINE_VERSION_1404.pdf

McAuley, A., Matheson, C. & Robertson, J.R. (2022). From the clinic to the street: the changing role of benzodiazepines in the Scottish overdose epidemic, *International Journal of Drug Policy, 100*(103512), 0955-33959. https://doi.org/10.1016/j.drugpo.2021.103512

McKenzie-McHarg, K., Ayers, S., Ford, E., Horsch, A. *et al.* (2015). Post-traumatic stress disorder following childbirth: An update of current issues and recommendations for future research. *Journal of Reproductive and Infant Psychology, 33*(3), 219–237. https://doi.org/10.1080/02646838.2015.1031646

Mekonnen, A.G., Yehualashet, S.S. & Bayleyegn, A.D. (2019). The effects of kangaroo mother care on the time to breastfeeding initiation among preterm and LBW infants: A meta-analysis of published studies. *International Breastfeeding Journal, 14*, 12. https://doi.org/10.1186/s13006-019-0206-0

Mikkelsen, S.H., Olsen, J., Bech, B.H. & Obel, C. (2017). Parental age and attention-deficit/hyperactivity disorder (ADHD). *International Journal of Epidemiology, 46*(2), 409–420. https://doi.org/10.1093/ije/dyw073

Milgrom, J. & Holt, C. (2014). Early intervention to protect the mother-infant relationship following postnatal depression: Study protocol for a randomised controlled trial. *Trials, 15*, 1–7. https://doi.org/10.1186/1745-6215-15-385

Mosley, P.E. (2009). Bigorexia: Bodybuilding and muscle dysmorphia. *European Eating Disorders. Review, 17*, 191–198. https://doi.org/10.1002/erv.897

Moyo, G.P.K. & Djoda, N. (2020). Relationship between the baby blues and postpartum depression: A study among Cameroonian women. *American Journal of Psychiatry and Neuroscience, 8*(1), 22–25. https://doi.org/10.11648/j.ajpn.20200801.16

Murphy, S.K., Itchon-Ramos, N., Visco, Z., Huang, Z. *et al.* (2018). Cannabinoid exposure and altered DNA methylation in rat and human sperm. *Epigenetics, 13*(12). 1208–1221. https://doi.org/10.1080/15592294.2018.1554521

Murray, S.B., Rieger, E., Hildebrandt, T., Karlov, L. *et al.* (2012). A comparison of eating, exercise, shape, and weight related symptomatology in males with muscle dysmorphia and anorexia nervosa. *Body Image, 9*, 193–200.

Musisi, S. & Kinyanda, E. (2020). Long-term impact of war, civil war, and persecution in civilian populations: Conflict and post-traumatic stress in African communities. *Frontiers in Psychiatry, 11*, 20. https://doi.org/10.3389/fpsyt.2020.00020

Nath, A., Murthy, G.V.S., Babu, G.R. & Di Renzo, G.C. (2017). Effect of prenatal exposure to maternal cortisol and psychological distress on infant development in Bengaluru, southern India: A prospective cohort study. *BMC Psychiatry, 17*, 255. https://doi.org/10.1186/s12888-017-1424-x

Nath, S., Russell, G., Kuyken, W., Psychogiou, L. & Ford, T. (2016). Does father–child conflict mediate the association between fathers' postnatal depressive symptoms and children's adjustment problems at 7 years old? *Psychological Medicine, 46*(8), 1719–1733. https://doi.org/10.1017/S0033291716000234

National Comorbidity Survey (NCS). (2017). Retrieved from https://www.hcp.med.harvard.edu/ncs/index.php

National Institute of Mental Health (2024). *Mental illness*. www.nimh.nih.gov/health/statistics/mental-illness

NCADV (2024). *Domestic abuse victim characteristics, England and Wales: year ending March 2024* Office for National Statistics. https://www.ons.gov.uk/peoplepopulationandcommunity/crimeandjustice/articles/domesticabusevictimcharacteristicsenglandandwales/yearendingmarch2024

NCT (2023). *Wellbeing & mental health traumatic birth and PTSD*. National Childbirth Trust. https://www.nct.org.uk/information/life-parent/wellbeing-mental-health/traumatic-birth-and-ptsd

Netsi, E., Pearson, R.M., Murray, L., Cooper, P., Craske, M.G. & Stein, A. (2018). Association of persistent and severe postnatal depression with child outcomes. *JAMA Psychiatry, 75*(3), 247–253. https://doi.org/10.1001/jamapsychiatry.2017.4363 JAMA

NHS England (n.d.). *Idea #1 Mapping the family and support network.* www.england.nhs.uk/mental-health/perinatal/perinatal-mental-health-resources/involving-and-supporting-partners-and-other-family-members-in-specialist-perinatal-mental-health-services-good-practice-guide/idea-1-mapping-the-family-and-support-network

NHS Wales (2022). *Postpartum Psychosis.* NHS Wales Perinatal Mental Health Network. https://executive.nhs.wales/functions/strategic-programme-for-mental-health/perinatal-mental-health/support-and-advice-leaflets/pnmh-support-leaflets/leaflet-8-post-partum-psychosis

NSPCC (2024). Parental mental health problems. NSPCC Learning. https://learning.nspcc.org.uk/children-and-families-at-risk/parental-mental-health-problems

Nwebube, C., Glover, V. & Stewart, L. (2017). Prenatal listening to songs composed for pregnancy and symptoms of anxiety and depression: A pilot study. *BMC Complementary Medicine and Therapies, 17*, 256. https://doi.org/10.1186/s12906-017-1759-3

O'Dell, L., Brownlow, C. & Thom-Jones, S. (2025). From 'refrigerator mothers' to paracetamol: why harmful autism myths are so common. *The Conversation.* https://theconversation.com/from-refrigerator-mothers-to-paracetamol-why-harmful-autism-myths-are-so-common-266075

Pawlby, S., Hay, D.F, Sharp, D., Waters, C.S. & O'Keane, V. (2009). Antenatal depression predicts depression in adolescent offspring: Prospective longitudinal community-based study. *Journal of Affective Disorders, 113*(3), 236–243. https://doi.org/10.1016/j.jad.2008.05.018

Perry, A., Gordon-Smith, K., Jones, L. & Jones, I. (2021). Phenomenology, epidemiology and aetiology of postpartum psychosis: A review. *Brain Sciences, 11*, 47. https://doi.org/10.3390/brainsci11010047

Perry, A., Gordon-Smith, K., Webb, I., Fone, E. *et al.* (2019). Postpartum psychosis in bipolar disorder: No evidence of association with personality traits, cognitive style or affective temperaments. *BMC Psychiatry, 19*, 395. https://doi.org/10.1186/s12888-019-2392-0

Persson, P. & Rossin-Slater, M. (2018). Family ruptures, stress, and the mental health of the next generation. *American Economic Review, 108*(4), 1214–1252.

Plant, D.T., Pariante, C.M., Sharp, D. & Pawlby, S. (2015). Maternal depression during pregnancy and offspring depression in adulthood: Role of child maltreatment. *British Journal of Psychiatry, 207*(3), 213–220. https://doi.org/10.1192/bjp.bp.114.156620

Prasad, D., Kuhathasan, N., de Azevedo Cardoso, T., Suh, J.S. & Frey, B.N. (2022). The prevalence of borderline personality features and borderline personality disorder during the perinatal period: A systematic review and meta-analysis. *Archives of Women's Mental Health, 25*(2), 277–289.

Qouta, S., Punamäki, R.-L. & El Sarraj, E. (2005). Mother–child expression of psychological distress in war trauma. *Clinical Child Psychology and Psychiatry, 10*, 135–156. https://doi.org/10.1177/1359104505051208

Quilty L, Dion K, Nixon A, Phillips J. *et al.* (2020). Social, financial and psychological stress during an emerging pandemic: Observations from a population survey in the acute phase of COVID-19. *BMJ Open, 10*(12), e043805. https://doi.org/10.1136/bmjopen-2020-043805

Rajmohan, V. & Mohandas, E. (2007). The limbic system. *Indian Journal of Psychiatry, 49*(2), 132–139. https://doi.org/10.4103/0019-5545.33264

Ramchandani, P.G., Stein, A., O'Connor. T.G., Heron, J., Murray, L. & Evans, J. (2008). Depression in men in the postnatal period and later child psychopathology: A population cohort study. *Journal of the American Academy of Child & Adolescent Psychiatry, 47*(4), 390–398. https://doi.org/10.1097/CHI.0b013e31816429c2

Raza, S.K. & Raza, S. (2022). Postpartum psychosis. In *StatPearls* [Internet]. StatPearls Publishing. www.ncbi.nlm.nih.gov/books/NBK544304

RCP & RCPsych (2013). *Smoking and Mental Health: A Joint Report by the Royal College of Physicians and the Royal College of Psychiatrists*. Lavenham Press.

Reed, R., Sharman, R. & Inglis, C. (2017). Women's descriptions of childbirth trauma relating to care provider actions and interactions. *BMC Pregnancy and Childbirth, 17*, 21. https://doi.org/10.1186/s12884-016-1197-0

Reissland, N., Aydin, E., Francis, B. & Exley, K. (2014). Laterality of foetal self-touch in relation to maternal stress. *Laterality, 20*(1), 82–94. https://doi.org/10.1080/1357650X.2014.920339

Robertson, E. (2024). Do you sing lullabies to your baby? Here's why you should! *Bump, Baby & You*. www.bumpbabyandyou.co.uk/baby/do-you-sing-lullabies-to-your-baby-heres-why-you-should

Ross, L.E., McQueen, K., Vigod, S. & Dennis, C-L. (2011). Risk for postpartum depression associated with assisted reproductive technologies and multiple births: A systematic review. *Human Reproduction Update, 17*(1), 96–106. https://doi.org/10.1093/humupd/dmq025

Sanfilippo, K.R.M., McConnell, B., Cornelius, V., Darboe, B. *et al.* (2019). A study protocol for testing the feasibility of a randomised stepped wedge cluster design to investigate a Community Health Intervention through Musical Engagement (CHIME) for perinatal mental health in The Gambia. *Pilot and Feasibility Studies, 5*, 124 https://doi.org/10.1186/s40814-019-0515-5

Sanflippo, K.R.M., Stewart, L. & Glover, V. (2021). How music may support perinatal mental health: An overview. *Archives of Women's Mental Health, 24*, 831–839. https://doi.org/10.1007/s00737-021-01178-5

Saxbe, D.E., Edelstein, R.S., Lyden, H.M., Wardecker, B.M. Chopik, W.J. & Moors, A.C. (2017). Fathers' decline in testosterone and synchrony with partner testosterone during pregnancy predicts greater postpartum relationship investment. *Hormones and Behavior, 90*, 39–47. https://doi.org/10.1016/j.yhbeh.2016.07.005

Scelza, B.A. & Hinde, K. (2019). Crucial contributions: A biocultural study of grandmothering during the perinatal period. *Human Nature, 30*(4), 371–397. https://doi.org/10.1007/s12110-019-09356-2

Shah, Y. (2025, 7 February). Harm OCD: Signs, symptoms, and treatment. NOCD. www.treatmyocd.com/blog/what-is-harm-ocd-guide-to-ocd-subtype

Sidebottom, A.C., Harrison, P.A., Godecker, A. & Kim, H. (2012). Validation of the Patient Health Questionnaire (PHQ)-9 for prenatal depression screening. *Archives of Women's Mental Health, 15*(5), 367–374. https://doi.org/10.1007/s00737-012-0295-x

Siegel, R.S. & Brandon, A.R. (2014). Adolescents, pregnancy, and mental health. *Journal of Pediatric and Adolescent Gynecology, 27*(3), 138–150. https://doi.org/10.1016/j.jpag.2013.09.008

Simpson, A. (2020). Commentary: Caring for a violent relative with severe mental illness: A qualitative study. *Journal of Research in Nursing, 25*, 8. https://doi.org/10.1177/1744987120938

Singh, S., Roy, D., Sinha, K., Parveen, S., Sharma, G. & Joshi, G. (2020). Impact of COVID-19 and lockdown on mental health of children and adolescents: A narrative review with recommendations. *Psychiatry Research, 293*, 113429. https://doi.org/10.1016/j.psychres.2020.113429

Stepp, S.D., Whalen, D.J., Pilkonis, P.A., Hipwell, A.E. & Levine, M.D. (2012). Children of mothers with borderline personality disorder: Identifying parenting behaviors as potential targets for intervention. *Personality Disorders, 3*(1), 76–91. https://doi.org/10.1037/a0023081

Stidham Hall, K., Beauregard, J.L., Rentmeester, S.T., Livingston, M. & Harris, K.M. (2019). Adverse life experiences and risk of unintended pregnancy in adolescence and early adulthood: Implications for toxic stress and reproductive health. *SSM – Population Health, 7*, 100344. https://doi.org/10.1016/j.ssmph.2018.100344

Stuijfzand, S., Garthus-Niegel, S. & Horsch, A. (2020). Parental birth-related PTSD symptoms and bonding in the early postpartum period: A prospective population-based cohort study. *Frontiers in Psychiatry, 11*, 570727.

Teng, E. & Steinbacher, D.M. (2013). Repair of the cocaine-induced cleft palate using the modified double-opposing z-plasty. *The Cleft Palate Craniofacial Journal, 50*(4), 494-497. https://doi.org/10.1597/11-178

Toh, R.K.C. & Shorey, S. (2022). Experiences and needs of women from ethnic minorities in maternity healthcare: A qualitative systematic review and meta-aggregation. *Women and Birth, 36*(1), 30–38. https://doi.org/10.1016/j.wombi.2022.06.003

Tommy's (n.d.). Obsessive compulsive disorder in pregnancy. www.tommys.org/pregnancy-information/im-pregnant/mental-wellbeing/obsessive-compulsive-disorder

Trevarthen, C. & Aitken, K.J. (2001). Infant intersubjectivity: Research, theory, and clinical applications. *Journal of Child Psychology and Psychiatry, 42*(1), 3–48.

Usta, J., Murr, H. & El-Jarrah, R. (2021). COVID-19 lockdown and the increased violence against women: Understanding domestic violence during a pandemic. *Violence and Gender, 8*(3), 113–139. http://doi.org/10.1089/vio.2020.0069

Vasiliu, O. (2023). At the crossroads between eating disorders and body dysmorphic disorders: The case of bigorexia nervosa. *Brain Sciences, 13*(9), 1234. https://doi.org/10.3390/brainsci13091234

Verstraeten, B.S.E., Elgbeili, G., Hyde, A., King, S. & Olson. D.M. (2021). Maternal mental health after a wildfire: effects of social support in the Fort McMurray Wood Buffalo Study. *Canadian Journal of Psychiatry, 66*(8), 710–718. https://doi.org/10.1177/0706743720970859

Vischer, L.C., Heun, X., Steetskamp, J., Hasenburg, A. & Skala, C. (2020). Birth experience from the perspective of the fathers. *Archives of Gynecology and Obstetrics, 302*, 1297–1303.

Wang, J., Zhou, Y., Qian, W., Zhou, Y., Han, R. & Zhengkui, L. (2021). Maternal insomnia during the COVID-19 pandemic: Associations with depression and anxiety. *Social Psychiatry and Psychiatric Epidemiology, 56*, 1477–1485. https://doi.org/10.1007/s00127-021-02072-2

Wee, K.Y., Skouteris, H., Pier, C., Richardson, B. & Milgrom, J. (2011). Correlates of ante- and postnatal depression in fathers: A systematic review. *Journal of Affective Disorders, 130*(3), 358–377. https://doi.org/10.1016/j.jad.2010.06.019

Wei, S.Q., Bilodeau-Bertrand, M., Liu, S. & Auger, N. (2021). The impact of COVID-19 on pregnancy outcomes: A systematic review and meta-analysis. *CMAJ, 193*(16), E540–E548. https://doi.org/10.1503/cmaj.202604

Wendell, A.D. (2013). Overview and epidemiology of substance abuse in pregnancy. *Clinical Obstetrics and Gynecology, 56*(1), 91–96. https://doi.org/10.1097/GRF.0b013e31827feeb9

Whooley, M., Avins, A., Miranda, J. & Browner, W.S. (1997). Case-finding instruments for depression: Two questions are as good as many. *Journal of General Internal Medicine, 12*, 439–45. https://doi.org/10.1046/j.1525-1497.1997.00076.x

Williams, M. (2020). Fathers Reaching Out Why Dads Matter: 10 years of findings on the importance of fathers' mental health in the perinatal period. https://maternalmentalhealthalliance.org/media/filer_public/20/bf/20bf5bef-ca4d-4601-9842-fdcc5b09c6f8/why_dads_matter.pdf

World Health Organization (WHO). (2001, 28 September). The World Health Report 2001: Mental health disorders affect one in four people [Press release]. www.who.int/news/item/28-09-2001-the-world-health-report-2001-mental-disorders-affect-one-in-four-people

World Health Organization (2023). Maternal Mortality Report. https://www.who.int/news-room/fact-sheets/detail/maternal-mortality

Zacharia, A., Lever Taylor, B., Sweeney, A., Morant, N., Howard, L.M. & Johnson, S. (2020). Mental health support in the perinatal period for women with a personality disorder diagnosis: A qualitative study of women's experiences. *Journal of Personality Disorders, 34*, 482.

Zhou, D., Li, X. & Su, Y. (2021). The impacts of education on domestic violence: Evidence from China. *Applied Economics, 53*(58), 6702–6720. https://doi.org/10.1080/00036846.2021.1937504

Subject Index

Author index